The people who work on books are like sports teams, medical teams, or fitness groups, working together in a team

D0482832

ACKNOWLEDGEMENTS

effort to achieve their best. Here are the key players on this book's team and their positions. This is but one of the ways that I can thank each of them for playing, for scoring, for taking the manuscript and making it better. From the depths of that place that links the mind and the body—mine with theirs— I thank each of you.

THE CAPTAIN: Shawn Lani, editor, designer, and compatriot. Ardis Bow, graphic design.

THE POWER FORWARDS: Erkki Lappi, Jeff Black, Burt Birnbaum, Raimo Siurua, and Ed Burke. They called the plays.

THE POWER GUARDS: Syd Winlock and Tom Raynor, who cleared the path for me.

THE ATHLETES: Melissa McKenzie, John Urys, John Taylor, Kim and John Fehir, George Parrott, Roy Benson, and Alice Bradyshaw. They trained with me and/or field-tested this information.

THE PLAYERS & FANS: Lauren Bergen, Albert Hardaker, and everyone else who is now using a heart rate monitor or who, because of this book, has decided to take the steps to link their mind and heart to achieve their best.

THE COACHES: Mark Allen, Owen Anderson, Ray Browning, Beth Kirkpatrick, David Martin, Lyle Nelson, Irv Ray, Rob Sleamaker, and Dr. Massimo Testa. They have contributed their expert advice, and we're all the better for it.

THE TEAM DOCTOR: Last, but certainly not least, Donna Lee, the editor's editor, who performed corrective surgery, amputations, and transplants as needed.

You've been a great team—thank-you all for playing.

FOREWORD

Imagine having a miniature electronic device that lets you know how hard you are working, so that you maximize your training time and race more consistently in competition. This device is out there right now; it is the heart rate monitor.

eart rate monitors have brought high-tech biofeedback training into the reach of almost everyone. Single-handedly, heart rate monitors have allowed athletes, coaches, and other ordinary people to develop sophisticated training programs, the likes of which were unheard of just ten years ago.

Your heart is the most important muscle in your body. In fact, it serves as a barometer for the rest of your body, telling you how hard you are exercising, the state of your emotions, and how fast you are using up energy. It pulls these physiological variables together, weighs them, and comes out with a signal that reports your overall condition. This signal is your heart rate, and the importance of this signal to everyone who exercises is why wireless heart rate monitors were originally developed in Finland. These devices monitor your heart rate with a degree of accuracy rivaled only by the most sophisticated sports medicine equipment.

From beginner athlete to Olympian to rehabilitation patient, many thousands of people have used and benefitted from heart rate monitors. The list of noted heart rate monitor users includes Greg LeMond, Joe Montana, Lyle Alzado, Bruce Jenner, Scott Tinley, Olga Markova, Matthew Brick, the Stanford Swim Team, the Washington Redskins, the Chicago Bears, the Toronto Maple Leafs, the Baltimore Orioles, the Winnipeg Jets, the Soviet Cycling Team, several US Olympic training centers, almost all divisions of the

Library of Congress Catalog Card Number:
92-62064

Eighth Printing: August, 1998
Printed in USA

Polar Electro Inc.
370 Crossways Park Drive
Woodbury, New York 11797

Lay out / Graphic design CIS / Finland

Additional copies may be purchased by contacting the
publisher or
Heart Zones
2636 Fulton Avenue, Suite 200
Sacramento, CA 95821
Phone (916) 481-7283
Fax (916) 481-2213
Website: www.heartzone.com

CONTENTS

FOREWORD,
by Ed Burke, Ph.D. 4

INTRODUCTION,
by Mark Allen 6

CHAPTER 1.
Meeting the Heart Rate Monitor 9

CHAPTER 2.
The Basics 18

CHAPTER 3.
Meeting the Heart 25

CHAPTER 4.
The Link between the Mind and the Body 32

CHAPTER 5.
The Keys to Your Heart: Your Max. and Resting Heart Rates 40

CHAPTER 6.
The Five Target Heart Rate Zones 54

CHAPTER 7.
For First-timers 70

CHAPTER 8.
How to Train with a Heart Rate Monitor 79

CHAPTER 9.
Special Conditions 86

CHAPTER 10.
The Heart Rate Monitor Diet Plan 96

CHAPTER 11.
Cardiac Rehabilitation 105

CHAPTER 12.
High Performance Training and Racing 113

CHAPTER 13.
The History of the Heart Rate Monitor 124

CHAPTER 14.
Live a Longer and Happier Life 130

APPENDIX A:
List of Heart Rate Formulas 135

APPENDIX B:
Max HR and Max VO2 Correlation 138

US Air Force, Army, Navy, and Marines, NASA astronauts (who use them while on their treadmills in space), Johns Hopkins University, and many heart institutes and hospitals internationally.

In many ways, training with a heart rate monitor is like having a portable, full-time coach attached to your body. Heart rate monitors take the guesswork out of training intensity and serve as excellent guides for those times when you need to accurately evaluate your performance and adjust your training regimen.

Sally Edwards is an athlete and coach who has gone through the varied experiences of training and competition—the planning, training, suffering, and joy of winning. What she offers in this book is practical. It works. We can take it out the next day and use it.

This book is written for those Sally cannot reach in person, and every effort has been made to describe the body's responses to training in terms that can be understood by everyone. This book contains the full range of her lectures and thoughts and the figures she uses to illustrate them. Here in one place is virtually all the scientific and practical knowledge the reader needs to know about heart rate training and monitors, reported by Sally from her own experiences, from the scientific literature, and from the experiences of such champion athletes and coaches as Mark Allen, Lyle Nelson, Ray Browning, and Roy Benson.

I can think of only one problem that this book creates—the individuals who read and study it are sure to have an unfair advantage over their competitors who haven't.

EDMUND R. BURKE, PH.D.
Colorado Springs, Colorado
August 1, 1992

INTRODUCTION

Each year there is another product or training technique that is supposed to turn even the most mediocre athlete into the next Greg LeMond. I admit, I've tried quite a few of them myself, from a simple carbo load drink to exhaustive VO2 Max/anaerobic threshold testing devices to all varieties of disc and three-, four-, and bladedspoke wheels. The one item out of all my years of testing that hasn't been dropped is my heart rate monitor.

bout seven or eight years ago, I hooked up with a friend who had done extensive work with a heart rate monitor in a lab and on the roads. He explained the basics of training with one and told me to give it a try for a month and see what I thought. At first having this beeping contraption strapped to my chest for every run and every bike ride seemed to take a lot of the spontaneity out of my training. When my friends would sprint for a city limit sign, I had to hang back so that the monitor didn't start sounding off that my heart rate was too high. At the time I thought I was missing out.

However after a couple of weeks of feeling like a slave to a mechanical device, I started to see not only improvement in my speed at all heart rates, but also that my recovery rate was getting significantly faster. My monitor was becoming my best training partner. I was receiving instantaneous and unbiased feedback as to what was really happening inside my body. I was starting to see that over- and under-training, speed, recovery, fatigue, and endurance were all correlating my perception of how I felt in a variety of workout situations with what my heart rate monitor was saying, I was finally able to put together a training program that made sense for my body.

I finally decided it was time to really test the results of the heart rate monitor training. I ran five miles on a track, keeping my heart rate at 155 beats per minute, and recorded my average per mile pace. It was around 6:45

minutes per mile. Then, at the end of that season I repeated the same test. My per mile time at 155 beats per minute had dropped to just over a 5:30 pace. That meant that I was running over a minute a mile faster at the same heart rate, the same intensity, just by training smarter with a heart rate monitor.

The principles of using a heart rate monitor may seem a little confusing at first, but if you read Sally Edwards´book, I think you will find that using a heart rate monitor will actually simplify your overall training program, giving it a more defined framework within which you can add as much creativity as you can come up with. You will train more effectively with a heart rate monitor, getting stronger and faster in less workout time.

I´ve used the monitor in almost every running and cycling workout over the past eight years, and I love it. I´ve stuck with it for two reasons. First, it´s easy to use and understand, as I´m sure you will find out by reading this book. For me, that is almost as important as its effectiveness, because no matter how effective a device or fine-tuned a program, I won´t use it if it is too complicated or takes too much time. The second reason is that it works. I´ve been able to keep improving my performances over the years without suffering the supposedly normal amount of burnout and injury that most athletes assume is part of the package.

Of course, heart rate monitors won´t do the workouts for you - you still need to put in the training. They also won´t keep you from doing crazy things that may hurt your body. But, if you are looking for an easy and extremely effective way to monitor your body, give you feedback that normally could only be found in a lab, and improve your performance by training smarter rather than harder or longer, then I highly recommend that you buy a heart rate monitor and give it a try.

See you on the roads. I hope you´ll have your heart rate monitor, because I´ll have mine for sure.

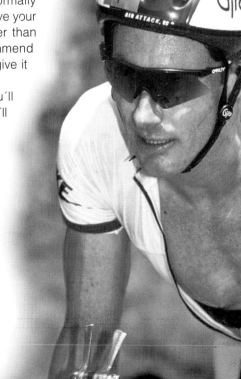

MARK ALLEN
Boulder, Colorado
July 13, 1992

Mark Allen during the 1992
Gatorade Ironman using a Polar
Vantage XL to win his fourth
Ironman title.
Photo: Lois Schwartz

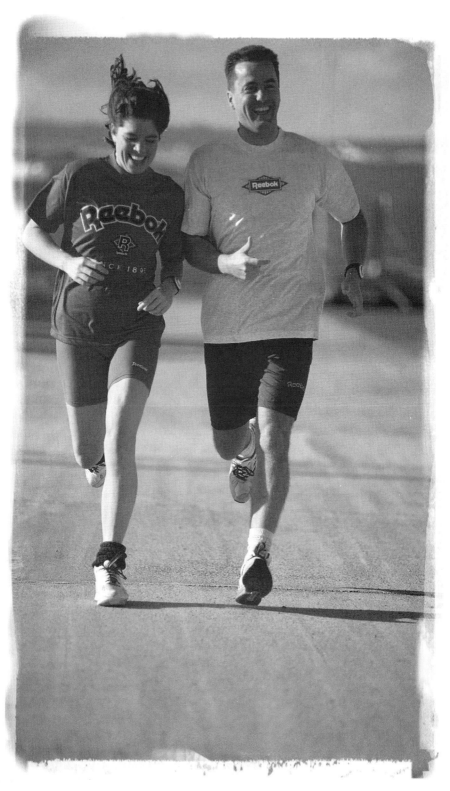

CHAPTER ONE

Meeting the Heart Rate
MONITOR

Forty years ago it was the stuff of comic books: a Dick Tracy watch that would monitor the wearer's physical condition. Ten years ago, heart rate monitors were the stuff of laboratories, where exercise scientists eagerly analyzed their athletes' cardiovascular conditioning. Today, heart rate monitors fit on your wrist and are as affordable as a good pair of running shoes and a warm-up suit.

asically, heart rate monitors provide biofeedback data—the key to regulating the intensity and quality of your workout. If you are merely guessing and going by your "perceived effort" (your inner sense of how hard you are exerting yourself), you lack hard data and are little better off than if you were completely uninformed.

Provided with useful biofeedback data, anyone can set themselves on a collision course with fitness. Think about it: there can only be one world champion, and yet there are millions of us who can have fun training like a champion. Being the best isn't as important as being your best, and heart rate monitors can help you get there.

Heart rate monitors work for anyone who wants to monitor their performance within safe ranges. They work for anyone who is rehabilitating from injury or from a cardiac condition. They work for anyone who wants to use biofeedback techniques to relax and recover. And they work for anyone who wants to lose weight or have fun.

For competitive athletes in their "I am training for..." mode, the heart rate monitor is a fine-tuning training instrument. For individuals more interested in fitness than competition, the heart rate monitor will maximize their exercising time and effort. This means that you can train less and benefit more from your workouts.

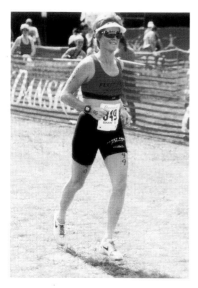

Every workout and every race, I use a heart rate monitor.

In this decade, athletes of the highest caliber have used wireless electronic heart rate monitors to win world championships. To many, heart rate monitors have become indispensable. Athletes such as four-time Ironman winner Mark Allen and Tour de France champion Greg LeMond avidly use heart rate monitors and have made them an important part of their training programs. They have long known the importance of understanding the mind's interaction with the body.

Some top athletes speak of "training secrets," alluding to seemingly magical training methods that escape the "common" athlete. After years of training, years of competing, and years of sports experience, let me tell you something—there are no training secrets. The entire range of knowledge in sports science is available to everyone. But technology moves fast, and when a tool like the heart rate monitor shows up, it's worth reevaluating your training program. Would farmers hoe fields by hand if you gave them tractors?

If you can precisely monitor and refine your training so that you maximize each and every individual workout, then and only then do you have a "training secret." It's a secret that can't be duplicated or copied, because it will be unique to you. Exercising at the best intensity or heart rate relative to you and your individual fitness goals would have been impossible without the introduction of the heart rate monitor. The reason is simple: heart rate monitors accurately measure your individual cardiovascular and physiological response to exercise.

But heart rate monitors can still be mysterious and even intimidating to the novice user. Don't be intimidated—be excited. Heart rate monitors are not only the most useful athletic tool to come out since digital watches, they're a lot of fun, too.

I found, as you will, that heart rate monitors are the single most important tool a fitness enthusiast can use today. The reason is simple: heart rate monitors directly link the mind with the body. Maybe you're presently of the "no pain, no gain" school of thought, and for you a good workout can be measured by the number of aspirin you have to take later that night. What you are doing is imposing your mind over your body, and that's not what you should be shooting for. Get your mind to work with your body. The information you get from a heart rate monitor will allow you to motivate yourself into a smart, efficient, systematic training program that will increase both your performance and your overall health.

MEASURING YOUR HEART'S PERFORMANCE

There are two methods available to determine your heart rate: manual and electronic. For years, people have been interrupting their workouts to put their fingers to their wrists or throats. By the time they stop, do the math and start up again, their training rhythm has been hopelessly interrupted. Electronic monitors are much more efficient and reliable and much less disruptive. There are two basic types of monitors: electrode chest belt monitors and photocell monitors.

Photocell monitors (also called photo-reflectance or infrared sensor monitors) measure pulse rate. A photocell or pulse-point unit uses a photocell sensor and a light source placed on the earlobe or finger to measure pulse rate. As blood circulates through a small arterial vessel, it disrupts the sensor's light pattern with each individual pulse beat. The data collected from this deflection of the light beam is transmitted to a monitor which displays the data as your pulse rate.

Strictly speaking, this type of monitor is actually a pulse meter, not a heart rate monitor, because it measures pulse rate, not heart rate. This may seem like a fine differentiation, but it is an important one. Pulse rate is a measurement of your heart's mechanical rate. That is, it measures how frequently your heart pumps blood through your arteries, causing them to expand. True heart rate monitors measure the electrical frequency of the heart, the number of beats per minute at which the heart is operating. Heart rate monitors use electrodes and measure the heart's electrical changes; pulse meters use sensors that measure the mechanical pulse from blood flow, which is then converted into a beat per minute readout.

It's also important to know that the photocell sensors used in pulse meters are not very reliable while out of doors because of the constant and sometimes dramatic changes in ambient light. In addition, they are rather sensitive to body movements and are not accurate at high levels of exertion. Finally, they are designed to respond very slowly to changes in heart rate. There are also some limitations on one's ability to program this type of monitor. The only real advantage photocells have over heart rate monitors at this time is price; they are relatively inexpensive, ranging from $40-$100. But to me, the loss of reliability and accuracy with photocell sensors is simply not acceptable—at any price.

Heart rate monitors, on the other hand, use two electrodes mounted on a sealed electronic transmitter that is attached to the chest with an elastic belt. These telemetry-based units pick up the electrical impulses from the heart and relay the information via an electro-magnetic field to a wrist monitor. They are extremely accurate (to within one b.p.m.) and can be programmed with numerous features that can help you train with greater precision. The correlations between the readings obtained by wireless heart rate monitors and readings simultaneously taken by electrocardiograph (ECG) hospital hard-wire monitors are extremely high. (The same is not true of the photocell monitors.) And, the prices for electrode wireless heart rate monitors, while not

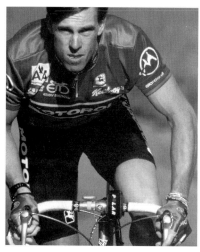

Some heart rate monitors can be attached to exercise equipment. Here the monitor attaches to the handle bar.

as low as for pulse meters, are still within affordability, ranging from $100-$400, depending on the number of features desired.

There are even some heart rate monitors designed to be used for working out in specific situations, such as on a bicycle, where a mounting device on the handlebars is used to attach the monitor for easy viewing. Some of these units not only provide you with your heart rate but will also tell you your training level (relative to your maximum heart rate) as well. In addition, the current and next generations of wireless monitors are being designed with consideration to looks—they are roughly the size of a wrist watch.

GETTING TO KNOW YOUR HEART RATE MONITOR

To get the most out of your heart rate monitor, you need to set aside about 30 minutes of uninterrupted time to read the instruction booklet that accompanies each unit and familiarize yourself with your new friend, the heart rate monitor.

For several years after purchasing my first heart rate monitor, I never took the 30 minutes of time that it takes to "meet your heart rate monitor." As a result, all I could do with it was strap it on and read the continuous heart rate display. I missed the opportunity to use the alarms, storage and recall, training zone limit, and time features. I used my monitor as a speedometer, not as a heart/mind biofeedback tool.

It took an airplane trip and an agreement with myself to spend the time to learn the special features that make a heart rate monitor such a useful piece of equipment. Whether you have had a heart rate monitor for a couple of years or have just bought one, commit yourself to learning all of its functions. All heart rate monitors provide a user's instruction manual of some sort. If you have misplaced yours, contact the manufacturer, and they will provide you with another.

The Polar Favor, a monitor model which only gives you your heart rate continuously, is one of the easiest heart rate monitors to operate.

The manufacturers have an obvious incentive: if your heart rate monitor is sitting in the drawer and not on your chest, their product hasn't really been a success.

The quick and easy way to learn the basics of all heart rate monitors is to demystify them. They may seem complicated at first, but you'll soon find that they are a lot simpler than they look.

There are only three components to all wireless heart rate monitors: a chest belt, a transmitter, and a receiver or wrist monitor. In fact, with the newer models of heart rate monitors, there are really just two components, as the chest belt and transmitter have been combined into one component with two parts, making for a very straightforward set-up.

The Chest Belt: This elastic belt holds the transmitter around your chest, is comfortable and easy to put on, and is adjustable for different chest sizes. On the inner side of the chest belt are two electrodes that sense your heart's electrical signals from the skin and relay that data to the transmitter.

The Transmitter: The transmitter either snaps onto the chest belt or, as mentioned before, is of one piece with it. The function of the transmitter is to send the heart rate data from the belt's electrodes to the wrist monitor or some other receiver via an electro-magnetic field.

Some heart rate monitors are waterproof.

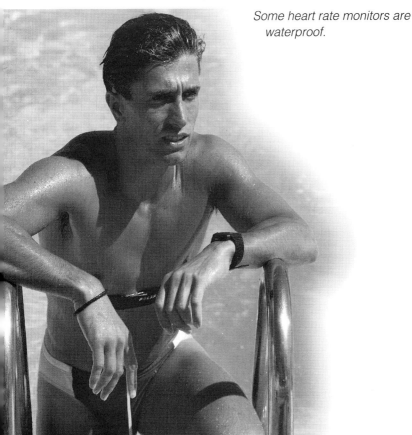

<u>The Wrist Monitor:</u> The wrist monitor looks like a wrist watch and functions as the receiver of the transmitter's signals. Different receivers give different read-out displays, but the basics are all the same. Following is a list of the various features.

HEART RATE: This number represents the number of heart beats in one minute (bpm) averaged over a period of time.

Time of Day: As simple as it sounds.

TARGET ZONE: This feature allows you to set high and low limits for your target training zone (TZ), generally in five beat increments. If your heart rate is below or above either of these two limits, a warning beep will sound with each heart beat and, in some models, the display will flash.

RECALL: This is the storage mode of a heart rate monitor which will give you read-outs of various aspects of your workout when you are done. Low-end monitors will store the amount of time you were above the low limit in your TZ; mid-range monitors will give you the time, in, above, and below your TZ; and high-end monitors will store your heart rate at specific intervals (such as every 5, 15 or 60 seconds), which you can use both to determine the amount of time you have been in each interval you set, as well as to graph the pattern of your heart rate's rise and fall.

STOP WATCH: Many heart rate monitors allow you to use them as you would a stop watch, but usually only when the heart rate function is on.

ALARMS: Many monitors also can serve as a standard clock alarm.

TIMERS: Some heart rate monitors allow you to set an audible timer that will chirp at specific points in your workout. A few models even have multiple timers. For example, you can set one timer to beep every three minutes to remind you to look at the monitor and check your heart rate and a second timer to sound off every 30 minutes at the end of an exercise interval.

STORAGE FILES: There are some top of the line heart rate monitors which allow you to store heart rate workouts in files, like you would on a desktop computer. At a later time, you can go back and recall the heart rate information. If you acquire the necessary computer interface and software, you can even download the data into a personal computer.

<u>Accessories:</u> There are a number of different items that can be used in conjunction with your heart rate monitor. For example, you can buy a mount for your bicycle, a harness to wear when swimming, an extra-large chest band, and computer software and interface equipment that allows you to print out your work.

When you are ready to actually put your heart rate monitor to use, follow these directions:

1. Snap the transmitter onto the elastic chest belt, if it is not already attached.

2. Snugly, but not tightly, hook the chest belt around your waist and pull it up to a point just below the level of your nipples and on or below the pectoral muscles.

3. Wet the two electrodes with water or saliva.

4. Wear the transmitter under your clothing if possible. If you must wear the chest band on top of your clothes, the fabric beneath the electrodes must be damp.

5. Set the wrist monitor so that it displays your heart rate and note your beginning heart rate.

Obviously, you need a heart rate monitor to use as we move forward. If you don't have one, stop now and read "Edwards' Buyer's Guide to Purchasing a Heart Rate Monitor" at the end of this chapter. There are over ten different manufacturers and 30 different models available. The chart should help you make an informed decision about the heart rate monitor features that best fit your needs.

Then, all you have to do is find the nearest heart rate monitor retailer—they are usually specialty sports shops, bike stores, or fitness equipment retailers. Make sure that you purchase your heart rate monitor from a store that can provide you with service and expertise on how to use your new training tool, with people who will be there for you if you ever have a problem.

Heart rate monitors are your friends, and like most close friends, it takes time to understand them, to get to know them, to break through some of the barriers that may keep you from knowing them better. A close friend of mine, Kim Fehir, a physician and triathlete, received a heart rate monitor as a birthday gift from her husband, John. He decided to buy her a top of the line model, because that is the kind of woman and athlete she is.

To this day however, Kim can't figure out how to use her heart rate monitor for anything but the simple heart rate mode. Kim continues to struggle with all of the features and is always saying to me: "Sally, I just want to know my heart rate. I just can't figure out how to set all of the zones and intervals and beeps. It is just too confusing." I say to Kim just what I am saying to you: your heart rate monitor is there for you. Look at it as a confidant, a motivator, a companion, and a supporter. In short, it should be your friend. Of course you'll always have people-friends, too. They can be a kind of "life rate monitor." You need reliable feedback when you are searching for your personal best, in fitness and in life.

One last hint for now. This book has been designed as an introduction to heart rate monitors for people of all interests, backgrounds, fitness and health levels, so every bit of every chapter that follows may not be tailored to your personal needs. But, since tailoring fitness to your personal needs is what heart rate monitors are all about, I'm going to give you a brief map of the course of this book, and from there you can choose to run whichever track best suits you.

THE FOUR RECOMMENDED TRACKS

Beginner/Fitness Enthusiast: Read chapters 1–9 and 13–14, and take it easy on the charts, graphs, figures, numbers, and expert advice and workouts. You can come back to these later when you are ready.

Dieter: As with the Beginner/Fitness Enthusiast, you should read chapters 1–9 and 13–14, but make sure and add chapter 10, "The Heart Rate Monitor Diet Plan" and give it special attention. You can read through or skip over the advanced advice, workouts, and figures, as suits your background.

Cardiac Rehabilitator: Chapters 1–9 and 13–14 will benefit you, too, but specifically take note of chapter 11, "Cardiac Rehabilitation." It was written with your needs in mind and was reviewed by physicians and specialists in the field; we all want to help you on your road to recovery. You can either skip or read through the various advanced figures and workout advice elsewhere in the book, as you see fit, but DO NOT try the advanced workouts unless your doctor recommends it.

Intermediate Athlete/Competitor/Pro: While you might find bits of the first chapters a little slow, there are bits and pieces of advice even there that you could put to good use in your training. Really, this entire book, with the exceptions of chapters 10 and 11, can apply to your training needs. You should even read the appendices on various heart rate formulas and anaerobic threshold tests; in high performance training, the more info, the better.

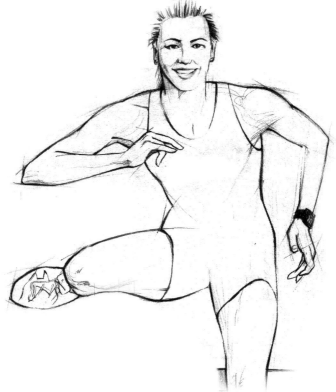

READY? ON YOUR MARKS, GET SET, GO!

EDWARD'S BUYERS GUIDE TO HEART RATE MONITORS

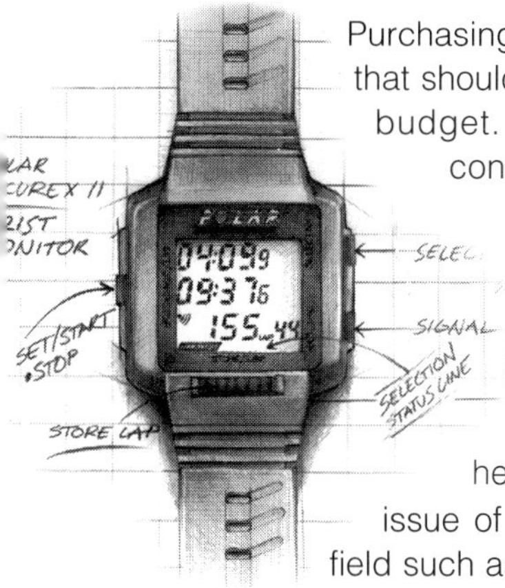

Purchasing a heart rate monitor is a very important decision that should be tailored to both your fitness needs and your budget. The first step, therefore, is to determine the consumer "need" category into which you best fit. You then can determine the features that are most necessary for your category and select the brand and model of heart rate monitor based on those features.

Please note that specific brands and models of heart rate monitors are not listed here, for the following two reasons. First, there is the issue of "datedness." In a fast-moving, high technology field such as the heart rate monitor industry, new models are released faster than new books are, and many models (or companies) that I might list here could be off the shelves before this book reached your hands. Second, there is also the issue of "universality." People around the world use heart rate monitors, but heart rate monitors around the world do not go by the same names. Therefore, I suggest you look to buy your heart rate monitor based upon your needs and its features, as I've outlined below.

NOTE: (The same four categories used above to describe the readers of this book should pretty closely fit the buyers of heart rate monitors, so they have been used in the following chart.)

| Features | Consumer Category: **x** = Necessary **o** = Optional | | | |
	Beginner	Cardiac Rehab	Dieter	Athlete/PRO
ECG Wireless	x	x	x	x
Time of Day	o	o	o	x
Stop Watch	x	x	x	x
Target Zone	x	x	x	x
Water resistant	o	x	x	x
Memory	o	o	o	x
Interval Timer	o	o	o	x
Computer Storage	o	o	o	x
PC Interface	o	o	o	x

CHAPTER TWO

SOME
BASICS

There are few basics, some tips and some terms, you need to pick up along the road when using a heart rate monitor in your training. Here they are...

1. Your chest belt usually needs a little assistance to get a reading because it relies on a certain amount of dampness for conductivity. Before you pull the belt up to its position below your pectoral muscles, wet the place where the electrodes are reading the information. Take water, saline solution (contact lens solution works really well), or saliva and moisten the area and then position the chest belt. Saliva actually works the best because of its high conductivity.

2. If you are getting a series of misreads, check to see that your chest belt is tight. A loose chest belt acts like an intermittent electrical connection causing misreads.

3. In the face of the heart rate monitor window, when the monitor is receiving a signal, a heart symbol flashes at the same rate as your heart beat. To test this, take your belt off and rub the inside location of the electrode contact and note that the flashing corresponds with the speed of your rubbing.

4. The transmitter emits a fairly weak signal to the wrist monitor, so interference from more powerful airwaves (from other exercise equipment to airplanes!) is not uncommon. The good news is that interference is usually quite brief and while misreads can be confusing, there is no reason to take them particularly seriously.

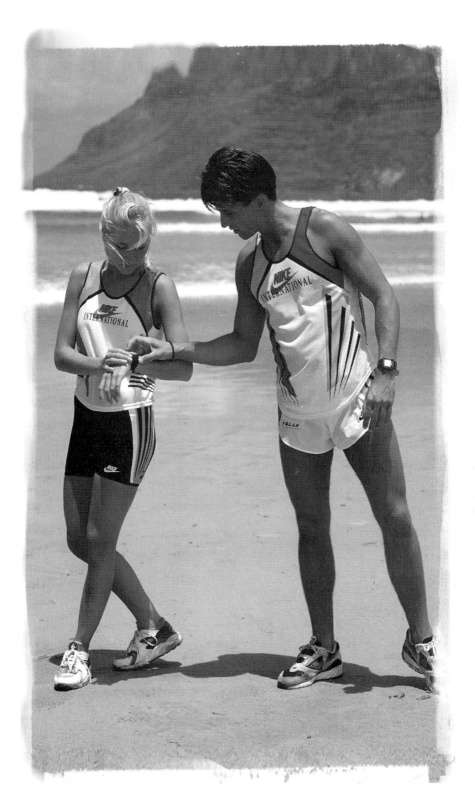

5. If you are outside wondering, do this simple test. Take off your transmitter or belt and look to see if the heart symbol continues to pulsate. If it is, then some other source is transmitting and your monitor is receiving that signal.

COMMONLY ASKED QUESTIONS

Question: I have worn my heart rate monitor enough so that I know my heart rate, so why should I keep on wearing it?

Answer: Your sense of perceived exertion might be highly developed, but perception and reality are too frequently very different. Can you perceive your level of over- or under-training and adjust? Can you perceive the effects of caffeine, humidity, fluid levels, changes in altitude, sleep, and emotional stress when you combine them together? Probably not, so continuing to wear your heart rate monitor is recommended.

Question: All I use my heart rate monitor for is to see my heart rate, so what else can I do with it?

Answer: The heart rate monitor is not a speedometer. It is not a tool to use to rev up your engines or to train to the point of maximal exertion. Rather, it is a highly powerful way of measuring, monitoring, controlling your entire program. The higher purposes of the monitor have to do with using it as a planning tool to design programs that work for you as an individual—systematically. Learn to use the heart rate monitor as your coach. Set the training zone limits and when you hear the alarm go off, think to yourself, "That's my coach telling me to slow down (or pick it up)."

Question: Yesterday my maximum heart rate while training was 187, and today it was 192; am I overtraining?

Answer: No, but you are developing a case of heart rate monitorosis. This is a condition that occurs when you become fixed on single heart rate numbers rather than heart rate zones. There are changes and repetitions in your heart rate readings on a daily basis, so you need to focus on training in your zones and notice the range of readings, not just any given one.

Question: I wear my heart rate monitor religiously, and I want to know if I have become obsessed with it.

Answer: If for some reason you don't have your monitor with you and this is enough to keep you from doing a workout, there is definitely something wrong. On the other hand, if you don't manage to wear your heart rate monitor regularly enough to get any benefit from it, you suffer from lack a of discipline. There is a balance between these two extremes that you need to achieve.

Question: Why is it that my heart rate monitor always reads such high heart rates?

Answer: There is a great deal of variation in heart rates between individuals of the same age, sometimes as much as 40 beats per minute. For example, my resting heart rate is 55 beats per minute, and I know of others whose are at 95 bpm. However, it has been noticed in retail stores that sell and service heart rate monitors that frequently men return them thinking they are defective because the rates are too high, while women return them saying that they can't get their heart rates high enough. That is the difference between perceived effort and real effort.

Question: Is the heart rate monitor a secret weapon that I can use to beat my competition?
Answer: Every athlete is looking for a secret. The heart rate monitor is not a secret or a weapon, but it is an extremely helpful tool you can use to enhance your fitness and performance.

Question: How do I calculate heart rates?
Answer: Read on through the next few chapters.

GLOSSARY OF FITNESS TERMS

Whatever world of work or play you find yourself in, there is always a slightly different lingo that goes along with it. The following list of terms are used frequently in the language of fitness and in this book.

AEROBIC. An exercise program easy enough to keep you from getting out of breath; literally, your muscles are kept "in the presence of oxygen."

ANAEROBIC. The opposite condition from aerobic; the exercise bout is so strenuous that the muscles are working beyond their capacity and are without sufficient oxygen.

BASE. A training term for the fitness level required to exercise for an extended duration without tiring..

CROSS-TRAINING. Working out in more than one sport simultaneously. Cross-training enhances overall fitness more quickly than single-sport training and also tends to provide more variety and stimulation. Also known as "multi-sport training."

ERGOGENIC AIDS. Any substance or technique, such as heart rate monitors, that can potentially increase athletic performance.

FITNESS THRESHOLD. The quantitative point, usually a minimum of three workouts per week, each of at least 30 minutes duration, that you must cross in order to achieve significant positive effects on your muscular and cardiorespiratory system from training.

HAMMER. A type of workout high in intensity and low in rest, usually in reference to bicycling.

K. An abbreviation for the word kilometer, as in a "5k" run.

KICK. The burst of speed at the end of a workout or race.

LEG. One stage or segment of a workout or race.

LSD. A training method which emphasizes long, slow distances.

OVERUSE. Training too hard, usually to the point of injury.

PACE. The average rate of speed of the activity.

QUALITY. Training which balances speed and distance.

RESISTANCE WORK. Training against something—a hill, winds, sand, or added weight—in order to overload a muscle group and grow stronger.

SPLITS. Dividing an event into parts based on time. For example, a bike split consists of the time from the start to the finish of the bicycling stage of a triathlon.

TIME TRIAL. A timed, simulated race, run over a known distance at a full racing effort, usually done solo.

TRAINING EFFECT. The term for the variety of physical and mental changes that occur when adapting to the stresses of workouts.

WALL. The barrier athletes hit when they are exhausted by the distance or pace of a workout and are barely able to continue to move.

EXTRA GLOSSARY OF HEART RATE TERMS

Sometimes, training can become really confusing. We are told to work out at a "percentage of max," but then we aren't told what the parameters are—oxygen/carbon dioxide ratios, lactates, pulse rate, heart rate reserve, or whatever. To keep anyone from feeling lost in the chapters ahead, we are going to preview the different kinds of heart rates or "cardiac frequency" measures. You don't have to memorize the following terms; they are just here for you to acquaint yourself with and refer back to if you have a need.

RESTING HEART RATE (RHR). This is the number of beats in one minute when you are at complete, uninterrupted rest. It is usually taken when you first wake up in the morning, before you lift your head off the pillow.

MAXIMUM HEART RATE (MHR). This is the highest number of times your heart can contract in one minute. It can be measured by taking a stress test or by using a heart rate monitor in your specific sport activity.

SAFETY HEART RATE (SAFETY HR). This is the heart rate that is prescribed for beginning exercisers—whether a walker, runner, swimmer, snowshoer, or a participant in any aerobic activity. It is also the term used in some cardiac rehabilitation programs in which physicians prescribe moderate, supervised training for recovering heart attack patients. This range is usually 60% (or less) of the MHR and represents the least amount of stress you can place on your heart and still receive a beneficial exercise effect.

KARVONEN TRAINING HEART RATE (THR). That heart rate recommended by the American College of Sports Medicine which uses resting heart rates in the formula to determine training levels.

HEART RATE RESERVE (HRR). The total number of beats (the specific heart rate range) that you have between your resting heart rate and your maximum heart rate. MHRR is the maximum heart rate reserve, and is sometimes called the "working heart rate."

RECOVERY HEART RATE (RECOVERY HR). This is the reduction in your heart rate right after you stop exercising. The higher your fitness level, the faster the drop in your heart rate. Total Recovery Heart Rate is the time between when you stop exercising and the time it takes for your heart rate to return to the pre exercise level.. A common Recovery HR measurement is one minute.

MAX VO2 HEART RATE (MVO2 HR). This is the heart rate at which you hit your maximal oxygen uptake effort. On the average, you hit your Max VO2 HR at 95% of your MHR.

ANAEROBIC THRESHOLD HEART RATE (AT HR). This is the heart rate at which you enter the physiological point where you are producing more lactate than you are able to synthesize.

EXERCISE HEART RATE (EHR). That heart rate which is optimum for the beneficial effects of exercising; your target heart rate.

CARING FOR YOUR HEART RATE MONITOR

You need to take care of your heart rate monitor in order to have optimal, trouble-free usage. If you follow these recommendations for its care, you'll probably be doing just fine.

1. Find out from your user's manual whether or not your heart rate monitor is water resistant; not all heart rate monitors are. If your monitor isn't, by all means, do not get it wet.

2. If your heart rate monitor is water resistant, do not operate its buttons underwater, as the water pressure can cause the receiver to leak.

3. Keep all the components of your monitor clean, and wipe off any extra moisture before you put them away. Never store your monitor in a closed, non-ventilated container such as a plastic bag or damp workout bag, where moisture and humid air can be trapped. Always store the unit in a warm, dry location.

4. If your heart rate monitor is not water resistant and you are a heavy sweater, wear a sweat band under the receiver or on your forearm just above it to keep the moisture away. Make sure your hands are dry when pressing the buttons to prevent moisture from entering.

5. Lubricate your transmitter snaps with silicon lubricant spray; it helps prevent corrosion if they are exposed to extremely moist or sweaty conditions.

6. If you have a two piece belt and separate transmitter, completely disconnect the transmitter from the belt after each use. This extends the life of the batteries and snap connectors.

7. Keep the elastic chest belt clean by rinsing with a mild soap and water solution. With time, the transmitter belt will wear out and cause disturbances or failure. Replacement belts are available from the manufacturer.

8. Don't stretch or bend the electrode strips of the belt, especially when storing, as it will damage the belt's conductivity.

9. Battery replacement for the water resistent models should be done by the manufacturer, as the rubber gasket seals that ensure water resistance will also need to be changed at that time and the unit tested for water resistance afterwards.

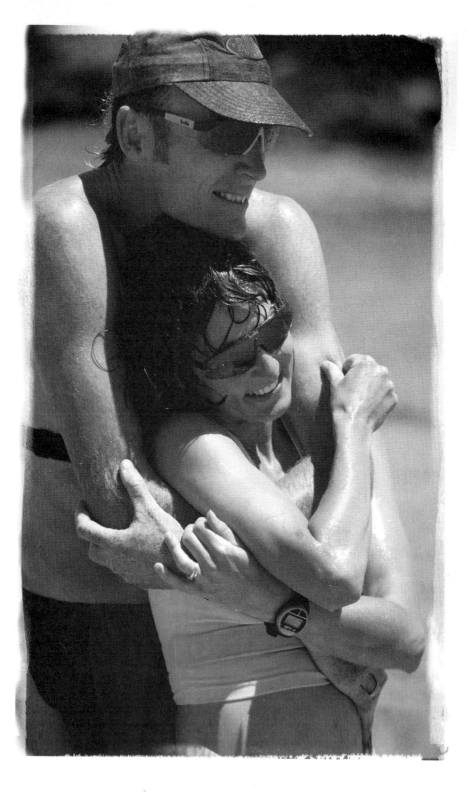

CHAPTER THREE

The word "heart" has come to mean a lot of things: courage, love, care, passion; grand concepts for a muscle the size of your fist. But as you will soon see, your heart is probably the single most vital, dynamic, and powerful organ in your body.

Meeting the heart

n many ways, the heart works just like any other muscle in that it has a specific job, a repetitive action it performs flawlessly day in and day out. It's that consistency and the ability to adapt to our physiological changes that makes the heart so remarkable when it is fit and healthy. However, it is possible for the heart, like any other muscle, to weaken and atrophy (get smaller) through lack of use, and this is a very serious problem of truly epidemic proportions.

After years of instructional efforts and research, heart disease remains the number one killer in the United States, and the American Heart Association has long listed smoking, high blood pressure, and high cholesterol as the major causes. Now however, there has been found to be another. In July of 1992 the American Heart Association took the strongest stand yet against cardiac atrophy when they added physical inactivity to their short list of major risk factors for heart disease. The implications of this should be very clear, but I will spell them out, just in case: Inactivity will cripple your heart as quickly as smoking, high blood pressure, and high cholesterol. Don't let it.

Here's the good news: there is absolutely no reason you have to give in to cardiac atrophy. Your heart can be developed and conditioned according to the same principles one would use to develop any muscle. Muscle development, the opposite of muscle atrophy, is called "hypertrophy," and it's what we are aiming for.

The average size of a sedentary human's heart (or the average heart volume) is 1.7 pints (800 ml). You can get an idea of its volume by visualizing a pint of milk and then imagining the size of your heart as over one-and-a-half times that amount. Your heart's mass will increase in direct proportion to the amount of aerobic training you undergo, up to 25% for some endurance athletes. Known as "athlete's heart," this cardiac hypertrophy occurs regardless of age and is similar to any muscle's reaction to an increased work load.

Don't think that just because you are not able to see your heart's size and condition directly that you can't get accurate feedback as to how your cardiac training is progressing. That's where a heart rate monitor comes into the picture. Heart rate monitors provide you with a window to your heart.

THE BIOMECHANICS OF THE HEART

Your heart is a pump. When it contracts, the heart pumps blood to the lungs on one side and to the trunk and lower extremities on the other. The heart is located under your chest bone, not all the way over in the upper left quadrant like we were taught in school, but nearly in the center of your chest.

The average heart weighs less than a pound, yet manages to efficiently pump blood with incredible force. If you measured the power from your heart's 40,000,000 beats per year, it would equal a force capable of lifting you 100 miles above the Earth. For someone of average fitness level, the volume and water pressure of a kitchen faucet at full blast falls short of what a heart working maximally can do. Seems like something out of the "Bionic Woman" or "Six Million Dollar Man," doesn't it? Well it's not science fiction; it's true. Your heart is a marvel of high technology that is standard human equipment.

We've been discussing the heart as a pump, but it is actually two pumps, each with two chambers joined together by valves. The heart muscle's right side receives blood in a chamber called the right atrium. The right atrium fills with carbon dioxide rich blood returning from different parts of the body, then pumps this same blood to the lungs out of a second chamber, the right ventricle. While blood flows through the lungs, it releases its stored carbon dioxide gases and reabsorbs atmospheric oxygen.

The left side of the heart receives this oxygen-laden blood in a third chamber, the left atrium. The fourth heart chamber, the left ventricle, then pumps oxygen rich blood out of the heart into the aorta and eventually into a multitude of arteries. The following figure shows the four heart chambers and how blood circulates through the heart's four valves:

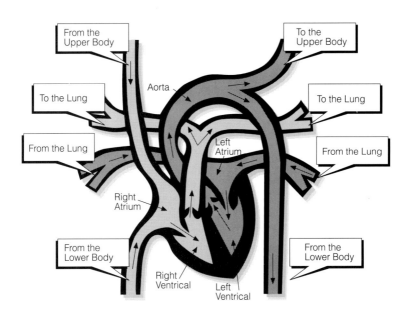

A working diagram of your heart.

The heart muscle's contractions are called heart beats and are generally measured in beats per minute (bpm). When the heart is not contracted and is at rest, blood is able to flow into and fill the chambers. Just prior to contraction, the valves that separate the different chambers open or close to allow the proper sequence of blood flow.

When the heart muscle contracts and blood flows out of the heart, it does so with a certain amount of pressure. When the heart muscle is at rest the pressure in the vessels decreases. The two different pressures, the high pressure at contraction (systolic pressure) and the low pressure during the rest phases (diastolic pressure) are the two numbers given when your blood pressure is measured. Let's say your blood pressure is 120 over 80 (120/80). The high number, 120, represents blood pressure immediately after a heart muscle contraction, when blood is flowing at its greatest pressure. The low number, 80, represents the blood pressure when the heart is at rest and the chambers are filling with blood.

Now, your heart rate, like your blood pressure, is generally controlled involuntarily, with normal resting heart rates ranging from 60 to 80 bpm. However, in highly trained athletes, resting heart rates in the low 30 bpm range are common, and when they are taxed to the maximum in strenuous exercise, rates according to Dave Martin, Ph. D.,as high as 210-250 beats per minute have been recorded.

If left alone, your heart regulates its own rate automatically, but there are a number of factors that can change the rate of your heart's contractions. For example, in addition to the circulatory chemicals (to be discussed shortly) which can raise or lower your bpm, there are also nerves that go directly from the brain to the heart which can signal a change in heart rate.

For example, think of an anxious moment: an unpleasant work experience, the last time you drove the wrong way down a one-way street, or walked out of a restaurant and forgot to pay. They're not pleasant thoughts (or experiences), but they will get your heart pumping faster.

OK, you don't need to dwell on it. Now breathe deeply for a moment, quietly relax, and think pleasant thoughts. (I'm not giving you any suggestions here, you have to think up your own; it's good practice!) Soon, whether you realize it or not, you will have lowered your heart rate and learned an important lesson: your heart rate can be, to a significant degree, controllable.

The rate of your heart muscle's contractions is controlled by a natural pacemaker, located in your heart's upper right atrium. This pacemaker is a bundle of specialized muscle tissues that receives regulating messages from your brain. If your cells need more fuel or more oxygen, the brain automatically speeds up the pump and increases blood flow.

The complete heart beat sequence is not unlike a musical rhythm. The rhythm consists of a sequence of electrical activities that occur in a specific set of patterns. These patterns are themselves translated into electrical waves. This sequence of activities starts with the valves opening and closing, continues as the heart muscle contracts and finishes during the post-contraction relaxation or pause. Throughout the contraction phase, blood is pumped out of the heart. During the relaxation phase of the rhythm there is time for blood to refill the chambers between beats.

This heart rhythm can be recorded on paper via the electrocardiogram. The height (amplitude) of the electrocardiogram's readings and the timing of the events can vary, but the basic rhythm looks as follows:

Heart Beat Intervals *(in seconds)*

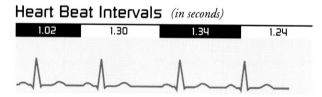

| 1.02 | 1.30 | 1.34 | 1.24 |

The heart or cardiac rhythm is scored by means of an electrocardiogram or ECG. An electrocardiogram uses two or more electrodes attached to the chest which are connected to an amplifier . These electrodes measure the transmission of electrical activity through the heart muscle. Voltage changes are also recorded.

Cardiologists and exercise scientists use electrocardiograms to measure heart rate objectively. The electrocardiogram provides a written record of the heart's electric events in sequence during the cardiac cycle. Electrocardiograms are used to discover functional heart abnormalities such as abnormal cardiac rhythm, problems with the conduction of electricity, changes in supply of the oxygen to the heart muscle, or any other symptom of tissue damage.

The difference between an electrocardiogram and a heart rate monitor is quite simple: an electrocardiogram gives a picture of the complete cardiac rhythm while the heart rate monitor only measures one part of the cardiac rhythm, the number of times your heart beats in one minute. Think of the heart rate monitor as a metronome and the electrocardiogram as the sheet music that your heart is writing.

Heart rates vary tremendously among individuals. Resting heart rates can vary as much as 50-60 beats between two people of the same height, weight, and age. They vary greatly between the sexes as well, with women averaging about 5-7 bpm higher than men, due to women's proportionately smaller hearts.

Fit people also have lower heart rates, some with resting heart rates below 40 bpm (known as "bradycardia" or low heart rate). Sedentary, unfit people have high resting heart rates, sometimes over 100 bpm.

Your heart rate is really an efficiency rating for your entire body. It can indicate the amount of blood your heart is pumping, and the higher the heart rate, the more energy is required for you to pump it. A heart with a lower rate requires less energy to pump the same amount of blood.

The heart is a "work now, pay now" muscle. This is different than skeletal muscles which are "work now, pay later" muscles. That is, the heart requires continuous fuel or "metabolic replenishment." For limited durations, skeletal muscles are able to contract without meeting their immediate metabolic fuel needs.

The heart's cardiac output is based on how often the heart beats per minute (HR) and how much blood there is being pumped (stroke volume or SV). The total cardiac output formula is pretty simple, Cardiac Output = HR x SV.

If the heart is weak, causing the stroke volume to decrease, it will maintain the same blood volume by beating faster. If you change either the HR or SV, the other factor will work to adjust itself accordingly to keep the cardiac output consistent. This is true whether you are resting or exercising. While the cardiac output increases with exercise, the HR and SV keep in close relationship with each other, each changing as the other changes.

A key indicator of your heart's efficiency is your heart rate reserve (HRR). Your heart rate reserve is simply the difference between your maximum heart rate (Max HR) and your resting heart rate (Resting HR). These terms will be discussed in more detail later, but understand for now that your HRR is simply the difference between your heart working at its maximum and minimum rates. If you can expand your heart rate reserve, it will reduce the chances that your body's demand for oxygen will exceed the supply.

The lower Resting HR which results from physical conditioning also allows a longer rest interval between heart beats. This means the heart ventricles, or chambers have more time to fill with blood. The more blood that fills the ventricles the more they are stretched, which means a stronger contraction and a greater ejection of blood.

Aerobic conditioning of any kind causes the cardiovascular system to strengthen and become more efficient. One easily observed result of such conditioning is a lower Resting HR. But this cardiac adaptation is reversible—when you lose your conditioning there will typically be a reciprocal increase in the Resting HR.

As discussed before, heart rates can be changed by other factors than conditioning, such as your emotional state. Similarly, you can raise your heart rate voluntarily in anticipation of exercise or a race. This is called "anticipatory heart rate increase" and is the result of the endocrine and nervous systems signalling for help. The body responds biochemically by releasing epinephrine and norepinephrine from the adrenal glands, key biochemicals which raise the heart rate. In one experiment, the heart rates of male athletes were measured at the starting line of a 60 yard dash. Just prior to the firing of the starting gun, before they took even one running stride, their heart rates had increased by over 150%.

The heart rate response to intense exercise is nearly immediate. The higher the intensity of the exercise, the higher the heart rate. Even in non-sprint events, heart rates for trained athletes of 180 bpm are common within 30 seconds of the start of a one or two mile run. After this quick increase in heart rate, further increases are more gradual, with several plateaus being reached during the run. This intense response is common in most sports with the exception of swimming. Swimmers' maximum heart rates are generally 10-13 bpm lower than that of other athletes, mostly because they exercise in the prone position and use upper body muscle groups (which are relatively smaller than the lower body muscle groups used in most sports).

There are ways to voluntarily control resting and submaximal exercising heart rates, but they require mental training. In one experiment performed with two groups of athletes, Group A were told to lower their heart rates while working out and watching their heart rates displayed on a monitor before them. Group B were also told to lower their heart rates while working out, but they had no direct biofeedback. The result was that the athletes in Group A lowered their heart rates 22% more than Group B. Clearly, biofeedback can play an important part in your ability to control your body.

One way of controlling anticipatory heart rate increase and exercising heart rate is to use a heart rate monitor while training and racing. In a workout, you can think down your heart rate by watching your wrist monitor and consciously focusing on breathing deeply and fully. You'll be surprised by your newfound ability to control a muscle that has been on auto-pilot for so many years.

I frequently train with friends with similar heart rate levels who share the same enthusiasm for heart rate monitors. Running on a beach recently, one training partner was frustrated that my pulse was always 10 bpm lower than hers. She asked if we could stop talking while we ran because she was going to focus on lowering her training heart rate, and she began breathing long and evenly. Within one minute she had consciously dropped her heart rate by five bpm, and by the last portion of the forty minute/160 bpm steady heart rate run, we were beat-for-beat.

My friend was elated by her newfound ability to control her heart rate and become a more efficient athlete simply by concentrating. The memory of her elation and that of others like her drives me to introduce heart rate monitors to nearly every new training partner, every business acquaintance, and to all those concerned about their physical and mental fitness.

DON'T COUNT YOUR HEART RATE

You've been told since you started working out to stop every so often and count your heart rate for six or ten or fifteen seconds and look at a chart or multiply to determine your heart rate. This is called the palpation method of counting heart rate because you take your fingers and palpate an artery in your wrist or neck.

Before the era of heart rate monitors, this method made some sense because there were no other alternatives. The gross errors from this method have been enormous, however. The first error is in the accuracy of successfully counting a heart rate when you are breathing hard, already tired, and wanting oxygen more than numbers. There is also a learning curve inherent in getting the hang of the technique, so beginners are oftentimes off on their counting, which can become quite a big deal when you multiply the figures out.

The second error is one of math—it's hard to multiply or read a chart when you are tired. Even though the charts make the math easier, they still require that you go over and look up the number, which can be a bit of a problem if you are not near one when you need it. Then you need to record that number the chart gives you so that you can compare it with the different training zones, requiring more math as well as your having memorized your target heart rates.

The third error comes from the fact that as you are taking your heart rate, you are resting, and your heart rate is quickly dropping and therefore not giving you the information that you want, the exercising heart rate. For example, aerobics instructors frequently have you stop, then they walk over to turn down the music, where they then say to get ready, and finally you start counting. During that scene, your heart rate can already have dropped 10-20 bpm, which can make you think you aren't working hard enough, because your heart rate is so low, when in fact that's simply not the case.

One study by Doctor James Rippe of the University of Massachusetts Medical School shows that 60% of the participants in aerobics classes could not take their heart rates accurately by palpation. The average error was 17 beats per minute—on the low side. This means that the majority of the individuals underestimated their actual training heart rates. They thought they were not training hard enough because of the method they used to take their heart rates, when in fact they were just fine. Rippe also showed in his study that as the intensity of the aerobics class increased, the error between counting heart rates manually and the actual heart rate as measured with a heart rate monitor remained just as bad. It really is a better idea to take your heart rate using a heart rate monitor rather than manually.

The first time anyone straps on a chest belt and wrist monitor, a funny thing happens. The person will look at his/her heart rate and say: "Oh, this is way too high. I can lower this." Sure enough, they consciously start to relax, breathe deeply, and subsequently lower their heart rate. Linking your mind to your body can be a very natural thing if you have a reliable biofeedback device.

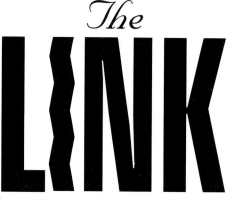

The LINK
Between the Mind and the
BODY

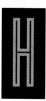

eart rate monitors are great biofeedback monitoring devices because they give a continuous reading of your heart's responses to various physiological variables: stress, caffeine, moods, images, feelings, thoughts, attitudes, etc. By staring at your heart rate monitor and focusing on your response as measured in beats per minute, you can learn a great deal about the cost of certain mental and physical states.

Sports psychologists have long been aware that the mind both consciously controls and unconsciously affects the body, and they have developed a myriad of concepts, theories, and philosophies to unleash athletes' mental powers and raise their performance levels. Many of the techniques may already be familiar to you, such as visualization, positive self-talk, and other means to control emotional states. Still, there are relatively few ways to interactively link the mind with the body and provide the feedback so essential for these mind/body techniques to work. Luckily, heart rate monitors are uniquely well-suited to provide the mind constant feedback about the body's best barometer—the heart—and that's what makes heart rate monitors such important training tools and why heart rate monitors are changing the ways people train and think.

Take the marksperson. To be successful, these athletes must mentally focus nearly every aspect of their minds and bodies. They learn to pull the

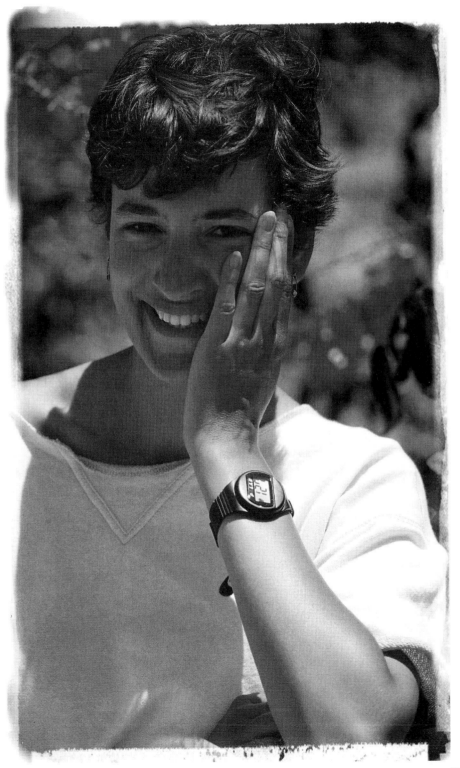

trigger between heart beats, at that split second of steadiness and calm, and the key to their doing that is their ability to train themselves to lower their heart rate at will.

THE INNER GAME OF BIOFEEDBACK

Heart rate monitors really have been an interesting addition to the sports psychologist's arsenal. Now, athletes that are under a tremendous amount of individual pressure, such as those in spectator arena sports, not only are being videotaped during games, but the psychologists are also recording the athletes' heart rates during play. Later, the heart rate readings are superimposed on the video screen so that the athletes' heart rate responses can be carefully analyzed.

Why are they going through all this? Because any number of factors can affect the athletes' heart rates and, therefore, their performance. If athletes were aware of the factors involved (i.e., minimal recovery time, negative mental feedback, distractions, or adverse weather conditions), they might be able to recognize potential problems before they had time to fully develop.

For example, if during a tennis match your negative self-talk convinces you that the match is hopeless, your heart rate will drop right in the middle of play in response to this psychological recognition of failure. Or, if your self-talk is stressful, but not necessarily defeatist, the anxiety could cause your heart rate to hover at a high, erratic, draining level, with equally fatal results for your game. Your coach, the heart rate monitor, could immediately let you know that your negative self-talk was adversely affecting your ability to perform. Ideally, you would take this information and, recognizing the problem, turn your mental attitude around.

This is the chemistry of emotions, the chemistry of anger, the chemistry of defeat, the chemistry of joy. All of these emotional states have a massive physiological effect on the athlete's ability to focus and perform. The best tennis players innately know this to be true, but those who don't have that sense already can be helped in developing it by using heart rate monitors.

The mind wants to control the body, and yet the body often has ideas of its own. The problem stems from your mind's lack of hard data: is your cardiorespiratory system really overtaxed, or are you just worried about tomorrow's mortgage payment? Your perceived exertion level is anything but reliable, especially at higher intensity levels.

In tennis, the majority of the match is actually spent standing still and resting between plays, and what players do during this time is one of the key components of their success. Players who use the time to quickly and consistently recover and keep their performance level as close to maximum as possible, have a staggering advantage over opponents who do not.

Premier sports psychologist James Loehr Ed.D., president of Loehr-Groppel Saddlebrook Sport Science, believes that what you think during periods of recovery is as important as what you do. High performance tennis players must learn their individual "ideal performance state heart rate zone."

This is defined as the heart rate zone which is just high enough for you to be excited about the play yet low enough that you are not overly aroused. For most players this is between 80-100 bpm.

Some tennis players actually play better when they are fatigued. This may seem odd, but once the heart rate monitor data are studied it all makes perfect sense. Fatigue can reduce nervousness and allow the heart rate between points to rise and fall as required by the game. As mentioned before, very nervous players get little to no rest, because as soon as play stops, the stress hormones emitted due to their nervousness keep their heart rates high, resulting in a linear heart rate. For example, if your between-point heart rates are recorded as 170, 165, 170, and 168, your emotional response is preventing recovery.

It is difficult (actually, nearly impossible) to simulate the emotional intensity of championship play in practice. That is why some of the most important training data comes from actual competitions. Still, you can use practice games as emotional and recovery training sessions, which will lead you to a better understanding of your body's physiological rhythms during competitive matches. Once you establish that crucial bridge between your mind and your body, you will discover that your competitive performance has always depended upon much more than training time, amount of sleep, and eating Wheaties. Any given match is as much a mental battle as it is a physical one.

Remember to pay attention to yourself, your mind, your inner voice, and all of your emotions. Sports psychologists have measured the performance effects of anger, negative mental self-talk, trying too hard, or not trying hard enough. The heart is amazingly sensitive to each of these conditions. Pay attention to your heart rate in each case—is it within your ideal performance state range? Measure it. Study it. Train using the data your heart rate monitor has provided you and focus your new control onto a more powerful game.

HIGH TECH AND HIGH TOUCH

In Megatrends, John Naisbitt predicted that the 90's would be "High Tech and High Touch." In this case, he's right. While undoubtedly a product of high technology, heart rate monitors are definitely "high touch." Through their intimate sensitivity with our bodies, they enable our minds to gently, methodically, respond to our hearts.

Heart rate monitors provide the means to accelerate the athlete's learning curve of self-understanding and fine-tune their ability to consciously adjust their body rhythms. Professional tennis players are using heart rate monitor data and the coaching of James Loehr, at Saddlebrook Sports Science, in Wesley Chapel, Florida, to do just that.

Loehr videotapes the individual championship performances of his players and analyzes their heart rates throughout their matches. He then correlates points won to heart rate levels to determine their individual ideal intensity levels. Once he knows the individual's ideal heart rate zones, he can create training programs that enhance the athlete's ability to perform within her/his range.

You, too, can determine your own ideal performance state heart rate zone. Use your heart rate monitor to monitor your performance throughout a highly competitive match, and then afterwards correlate your heart rate readings with your points won and lost. (A good memory and the cooperation of your partner will help here if you don't have the ability to videotape your match.)

Other sports could learn a lesson from Loehr's research. Take basketball players. At what heart rate do they make the highest percentage of baskets or the lowest number of defensive errors? If, at a point late in the game, the athlete's heart rate hovers too high for too long, they could be benched for a recovery break. Once on the bench, the players would be able to recover quickly using proven relaxation techniques. Yelling at referees, pacing, or sitting without a back rest certainly does nothing to calm the athlete down.

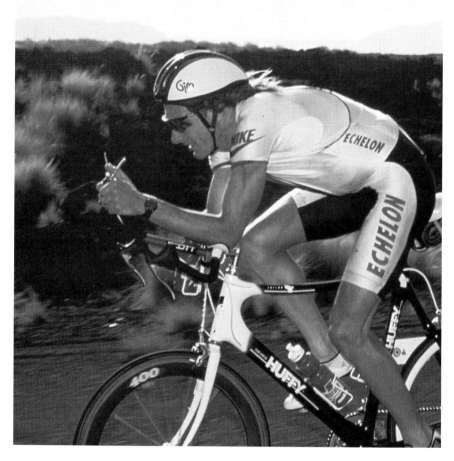

Mark Allen is affectionately known as the "Zen Master" because he uses the power of his mind to push his body to new limits. The heart rate monitor is his link between the two.

Players must learn to relax their minds, and focus on positive thoughts and visualizations, thereby unloading the mental and physical stress built up during competition. Once their heart rate drops, they could be put back in the game, ready to perform.

The athletes of the future will control their bodies and emotional states by using heart rate sensitivity. They will set their optimal heart rate levels and check their heart rate monitors often during competition to ensure that they are within their ideal heart rate zones. They will use heart rate monitor training to learn how to recover during their rest intervals. They will use heart rate monitors to determine when their level of fatigue impedes their ability to perform. They will understand the dynamic relationship between the mind and body—how one affects the other, and how both, in essence, are one.

SCHOOL KIDS AND HEART RATE MONITORS

"Ultra Physical Education" at Tilford Middle School is an example of what modern physical education can be, an opportunity for holistic education that is effective in bringing both knowledge and excitement to students' lives. In practice, this means that these "physical education" classes integrate science, music, math, computer science, health, stress management, home economics, and more with the education of the physical body. Ultra Physical Education is the union of the scholastic aspects of school with the body, using technology as the binding glue that holds kids' interests and guides them toward further exploration.

For students, one major part of Ultra Physical Education is learning how the body works by using heart rate monitor conditioning and testing. We have seen that not only are heart rate monitors and other technological devices key to enhancing students' ability to develop personal healthy lifestyle prescriptions, these tools also cause students' self-esteem to rise significantly just from being able to use them.

During each physical education class, the students train for a minimum of nine minutes in their target heart rate zone using a Polar Vantage XL heart rate monitor. Also each day, 12-18 students wear heart rate monitors set for each of their individual target heart rates throughout the entire class period.

At the end of the class, all heart monitors are checked back in, and the data is retrieved and stored on computer disks for later analysis. Records of the students' mile run times, recovery heart rates, and resting heart rates are all stored on data bases and downloaded to the computerized physical education report card system with all other information received during the term.

Parents may view their student's entire year's worth of data from physical education classes. Here is a sample print-out from a nine-minute run and the heart rate response during the test.

The documenting of students' heart rate data throughout their middle school years has proven to be invaluable in many ways. Students quickly learn proper pacing techniques, as well as how to determine exercise intensity levels in order to improve their levels of conditioning; basic principles of fitness are easy for students to see with the continuous feedback from the heart rate monitors. The effects of humidity, wind, different sports, and temperature provide students with hands-on math and science learning. And most significantly, the testing results comparing the fall to the spring show the majority of students having significant improvement in their levels of cardiovascular fitness.

Researchers concluded with a study published in the Journal for School Health (March 1989) that the students at Tilford Middle School were grasping advanced cognitive concepts, that they felt good about themselves, that they looked forward to physical education class, and that they intended to exercise in the future. We have not had a single student suspended because of drug use over the past five years, and fewer than two students per year over the past five years have received suspensions because of smoking.

By incorporating technology into the physical education classroom and providing quality daily physical education, this generation of students will have the chance to make healthy lifestyle choices. It is our responsibility, through tools such as the heart rate monitor, to help our children develop personal healthy lifestyle prescriptions, so that they will have the mental, physical, and emotional fitness and health to meet the demands of life beyond the year 2000.

Beth Kirkpatrick has been developing the Ultra Physical Education program as physical education teacher at Tilford Middle School in Vinton, Iowa, for the past eleven years. She encourages educators and individuals who would like to know more about the program to contact her. She can be reached by writing to Ball State University.

HEART RATE CURVE

Heart Rate
(Beats per minute)

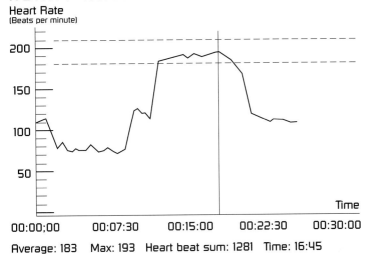

Average: 183   Max: 193   Heart beat sum: 1281   Time: 16:45

Beth Kirkpatrick's print-out of an 8th grade student during a one mile test

The reason we train is simple: to cause physiological adaptations to higher levels of athletic performance. That about sums it up. Sure, we train to control our weight, for emotional calm,

THE KEYS TO YOUR HEART

resting and

MAXIMUM HEART RATES

for the overall fitness, and for other personal reasons. But down deep, we exercise, we workout, we train, whatever you want to call it, because we just plain want to improve ourselves.

To truly improve our performance, we must coordinate and focus on all of the factors involved: frequency and length of workouts, type of training, speed, intensity, duration, and repetition of the specific activity or sport. How far can your performance progress? Who knows? There are countless factors that dictate your athletic limits. What really matters is your ability to achieve your personal best in a world where many give up before they even try. And a heart rate monitor can help you get to where you're going with confidence and efficiency.

Historically, coaches and trainers have required that all individuals do the same workout at the same intensity level, ignoring the individuality of athletes' adaptation rates and genetic abilities. Now we know that training is an individual matter and that individuals vary greatly. What is a high level of intensity for one person might well be below the training threshold intensity for another who is in better shape or who is genetically gifted.

Because of this, training needs to be assigned on a relative stress basis. That is, training intensities need to be set as percentages of each individual's maximum function that are based on the individual and their fitness level.

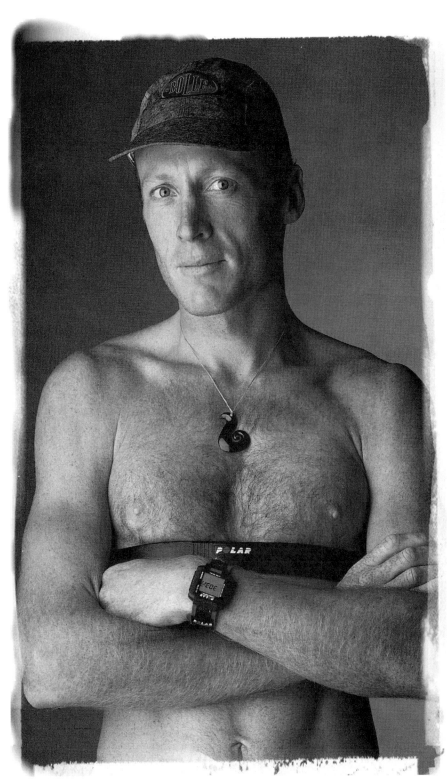

THERE ARE SEVERAL WAYS TO MEASURE TRAINING INTENSITY:

MAXIMUM HEART RATE (MAX HR): This is the heart rate at which increased intensity of exercise does not cause an increase in heart rate. The maximum heart rate number equals the maximum amount of times in one minute that your heart can contract, and this number cannot be increased; it can only be decreased by age.

MAXIMUM VO2 (MAX VO2): This is the maximum volume (V) of oxygen (O2) that you can utilize regardless of intensity increases. It is synonymous with maximal oxygen consumption, maximal oxygen uptake, or maximal aerobic power.

MAXIMUM WORK CAPACITY: The ability of a person to perform work. It is measured by metabolic rate, METs (the energy cost of the work), oxygen consumption, heart rate, and oxygen pulse. It is also called functional capacity.

LACTATE THRESHOLD: The point when lactic acid (a by-product of muscle contractions, more on this later) begins to increase faster than it can be shuttled or resynthesized.

HEART RATE RESERVE: The difference between your Max HR and your Resting HR represents your heart rate reserve. The greater the difference, the larger your heart rate reserve is and the greater your range of heart rate training intensities can be. There is no data to show a larger heart rate reserve means better performance.

Of these five ways of measuring training intensities, Max HR is the most logical measure for most athletes to use, because it is the only practical one for us to figure out on our own. To accurately determine maximum work capacity, Max VO2, and lactate thresholds requires expensive and sophisticated equipment. Sure, if you could do all of your training in a laboratory with electronic computerized gadgetry and recording devices connected to you, you could measure almost all of the factors involved in training, but that is simply not practical or economical.

Fortunately, exercise scientists have proven that all of these measurements are accurately related to one another. One's max VO2 and Max HR are predictably related to each other within plus or minus 8% above the 50% range; that is, when one is training at a given percent of their Max HR, they are at a predictable percentage of their Max VO2. This is true regardless of the sex or age of the individual. Here's how Max HR and Max VO2 compare:

THE RELATIONSHIP OF MAX HR TO MAX VO2

Percent of Maximum Heart Rate (MHR)	Percent of Maximum VO2 or Maximum Aerobic capacity
50	35
60	48
70	60
80	73
90	86
100	100

The term "maximums" often causes confusion among athletes unaware of the various maximums they could be referring to: heart rate (Max HR), aerobic capacity (Max VO2), or lactate buildup (millimoles of lactate). As you can see, there is no "one for one" equivalence between the percentage of Max HR and percentage of max VO2. Let's imagine that you are sitting in a chair at rest. Let's take your resting heart rate at it's 60 bpm. You took a Max HR test running and you found out that your maximum heart rate for running is 180 bpm. At complete rest, you are working at 30% of your Max HR. If we were to measure your VO2 at this same resting heart rate, it would be about 3.5 ml km-1min-1 which is about 10% of your Max VO2. That is, at rest you are using about ten percent of your maximum aerobic power while you work at 30% of your Max HR.

If you would like to know more about how to predict one from the other, that is how you can predict your Max HR if you know your Max VO2 or vice-versa, refer to Appendix B and there are formulas for this calculation.

As you can see, 70% Max HR is equivalent to 56% Max VO2. I frequently hear percentages tossed around as if they were identical for each of these physiological measures, but they certainly are not. If you are in doubt as to what "Max" we are referring to in this book, you can safely assume it will be Max HR and percentages thereof, unless I've clearly said otherwise. I urge others to distinguish among the many "Max's" and to use Max HR instead of other measures in all of their future coaching, clinics, and writings, in the hope that athletes will learn to use and refer to their "maximums" correctly.

THE AGE-ADJUSTED MAXIMUM HEART RATE FORMULA

There is a mathematical formula that allows you to predict your Max HR with some accuracy. It is called the "age-adjusted formula." Since it is not advisable for beginners or individuals in rehabilitation to take a Max HR test on their own, the age-adjusted Max HR formula can come in very handy when you're not prepared to pay the $100–$500 a physician-supervised stress test can run.

For women the formula is: 226 – your age = age-adjusted Max HR.
For men the formula is: 220 – your age = age-adjusted Max HR.

If you are 30 years old, your age-adjusted maximum heart rate is calculated as follows:

Age-adjusted Maximum Heart Rate   = 226 – your age
      (for women)   = 226 – 30 years
                  = 196 bpm (if you are 30 years old)

Age-adjusted Maximum Heart Rate   = 220 – your age
      (for men)   = 220 – 30 years
                  = 190 bpm (if you are 30 years old)

The numbers 220 and 226 seem to be the closest approximations of the average male and female Max HRs when rates are measured after puberty. This formula should not be used with children.

Empirical data leads many people to question this formula, however. For example, according to the age-adjusted formula, if you are a 25 year old male, then theoretically your Max HR is 220 – 25 or 195 bpm, but that is close to my Max HR, and I am a 45 year old woman.

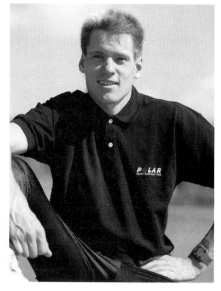

If you choose to use the age-adjusted formula, just remember that there may be some discrepancy. The age-adjusted formula will give you a ballpark guesstimate to work from, but if you want to exercise/train at your most effective levels, you should not rely on the figures the age-adjusted Max HR formula provides. A Max HR test, such as those described in the following section, is recommended.

Pauli Kiuru, one of the best triathletes in the world, trains and races systematically with a high quality heart rate monitor

TESTING YOUR MAXIMUM HEART RATE

As we have discussed, the accurate calculation of your maximum heart rate (Max HR) is crucial to the development of a truly effective personal fitness program. Although there are a number of mathematical equations that can let you calculate your Max HR, I've always been a big believer in verifying these numbers with actual performance tests.

The safest and most recommended method for determining your Max HR is to have your physician or sports physiologist give you a maximal stress test and health appraisal. Physicians will generally administer the test on a treadmill or exercise bicycle. The test will accurately, safely, and precisely indicate your Max HR, as well as provide you with other interesting data such as your Max VO2 and lactate thresholds. The cost for a stress test varies greatly, but they usually run between $100-$500 per test.

Now, obtaining a physician-supervised stress test may not always be possible, feasible, or recommended. The American College of Cardiology and the American Heart Association in a joint report question the value of diagnostic exercise testing in apparently healthy individuals. The authors of the report state that "exercise testing is of little or no value, inappropriate, or contraindicated" for "asymptomatic, apparently healthy women and men with no risk factors for coronary artery disease." Individuals at significant risk who are recommended to obtain physician-supervised stress tests are those with two or more major coronary risk factors and/or symptoms suggestive of cardiopulmonary or metabolic disease.

Two final warnings, one from the American College of Sports Medicine:

At or above 35 years of age, it is necessary for individuals to have a medical examination and a maximal exercise test before beginning a vigorous exercise program. At any age, the information gathered from an exercise test may be useful to establish an effective and safe exercise prescription. Maximal testing done for men at age 40 or above or women age 50 and older, even when no symptoms or risk factors are present, should be performed with physician supervision.

And one from me:

Do not take the following self-administered tests if you are over 35 years of age, have been sedentary, or for any reason are in poor physical condition and have not had a thorough physical exam (including an exercise stress test) and physician's release.

Heed these words well.

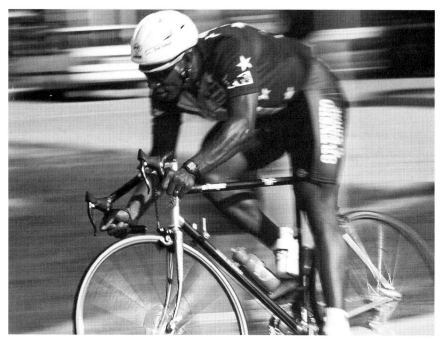

Anytime you take a maximum heart rate test, like cyclist Nelson Vails, you are pushing yourself competely for all-out speed!

MAXIMUM HEART RATE TESTS

Unfortunately, there is no way to increase your Max HR. Max HRs seem to be basically determined by our genetic backgrounds, and they do not seem to significantly change with training of any kind. The aging process is the only factor we've identified that changes Max HRs at all, and it does it in the wrong direction, unfortunately.

However, Max HR is dependent on the specific sport activity. Your Max HR in cycling will be slightly different from that in cross-country skiing, swimming, running, or aerobics. This means that if you cross-train, you need to take Max HR tests for each different sports activity. Upper-body sports activities tend to test between 10-13 bpm less than lower-body activities. Max HR for swimmers, for example, is usually 10-13 beats lower than tested Max HR for runners, in both fit and unfit individuals. For me, the maximum heart rate between my three sports varies sufficiently that it really does need to be taken into consideration. Check it out for yourself and see if it does for you, too.

The Max HR difference between upper- and lower-body activities is probably the result of the relatively smaller amounts of muscle mass in the upper body versus the lower. To establish the heart rate intensities for swimming or other upper-body activities if you don't take sport-specific Max HR tests, this 10-13 beat difference should be taken into account.

MAX HR TESTS: PREPARATION

The time of day that you take the Max HR test is important to your performance. It is best to take the test when the effects of ambient temperature (measured in degrees Fahrenheit) and humidity (measured as a percentage) combined together equals a value less than the number 160 (for Celsius, this combined value is approximately 100). For example, if it is 65 degrees Fahrenheit and the humidity is 70%, then the combined value of these environmental conditions is 135. For this reason, Max HR tests usually take place in the early morning or late evening (when you are not exposed to direct sunlight).

Time your meals before you take the test. Wait at least an hour after a medium to large meal. Some people find that it is best to have a small amount of food in their stomach prior to the test, while for others this causes cramping and stomach problems.

For any Max HR test to be successful, it should simulate what is called a "graduated stress test" in protocol. This requires that as the test progresses, either the pace, the surface incline, or the resistance should increase the amount of workload. Individual preference seems to be the deciding factor on which Max HR test you prefer. Regardless, they all require that you exercise extremely hard, to the point that you will be uncomfortable (that's a polite way of saying that it will hurt!).

Please note that while some muscular pain is expected with Max HR tests, if at any time you feel chest pain or have difficulty breathing, immediately begin to stop the test by reducing the intensity until your heart rate is below 100 bpm. Then, consult your physician before carrying out the test again. If your heart rate goes above the age-adjusted maximum that you calculated, then you need to be very cautious.

Finally, with all of the following tests, remember to both warm up beforehand and cool down afterwards. Knowing your Max HR won't do you much good if you are laid up with a hamstring or groin pull or worse! The proper warm-up and cool-down protocol varies from person to person and activity to activity, so I can't give you any hard and fast rules here, but the following guidelines may help.

The foremost things to remember are that the function of warm-ups and cool-downs is to ease your body's transition from a resting to an active state and back again, and that all of your muscles need to be taken into account. Many people remember to give their arms, legs, torso, and neck a good stretching (at least five minutes on either end of your workout is recommended), but they forget to warm up and cool down the most key muscle of all, their heart.

Each time you begin any strenuous exercise, you need to gradually increase the speed of your body's movements to bring up your heart rate to at least the lower limit of your target training zone before going all out in your workout. Likewise, when you complete your target training zone workout, you need to gradually slow down your movements to ease your heart rate down to the high end of your resting heart rate range, before you can consider yourself done and come to a full stop. For example, when I'm ready to go on a run, I start by slogging along slowly, then I pick up the pace to a jog, before I go full tilt into a run; I also do the reverse when I'm ready to cool down. Common sense applies here, as does your heart rate monitor. Use it to guide you through your warm-ups and cool-downs, as well as in your training zone workouts.

Now, for the tests...

MAX HR TESTS: GENERAL SPORTS ACTIVITIES

1. The All-Out Test: Exercise at the highest pace that you can maintain for two to four minutes such that towards the end of the time period, your heart rate no longer increases. This test should be repeated again after a ten minute rest. Max HR is usually the highest heart rate registered toward the end of this period.

2. The Race Test: Begin a race event of short to moderate distance. In the last 1-2 minutes, reach down deep and push yourself hard. Your Max HR will usually be the highest heart rate registered toward the end of this period.

3. The 800 Meter Test: Run (ski, bike, etc.) 800 meters (two laps around a high school or college track) at 85-90% of your age-adjusted Max HR. Jog (ski, bike, etc.) at an easier pace for 30 seconds. Then, run (ski, bike, etc.) a second 800 meters at top speed. Your Max HR is usually the highest heart rate registered toward the end of this period.

MAX HR TESTS: RUNNING

1. The 12 Minute Test: This is a test that can be repeated as needed to determine improvement in your conditioning. Ken Cooper in his original book Aerobics developed the procedures for the 12 Minute Run Test. After warming up, run at an even pace for at least ten minutes and then at an all-out pace for the last two minutes. Measure the total distance covered during the 12 minutes. As fitness improves, you should be able to cover a longer distance in the same amount of time. Max HR is usually the highest heart rate registered toward the end of this period.

2. The 1-Mile Test: Run as fast as you can for one mile or four laps around a track. Keep track of the total elapsed time during the one mile run, as you should be able to improve your time as you become more fit. Your Max HR will be the highest heart rate registered toward the end of this period.

3. Hill Repeat Test: Locate a "90 second hill," that is, a relatively steep hill that takes you about 90 seconds to run up. After you warm up, run four times up as hard as you can, then run or jog down the hill to recover to your pre-test heart rate. The Max HR is usually the highest heart rate registered toward the end of this period.

4. Graduated Test: Take your best one mile time or, if you don't know it, predict it with the help of a pace chart. Go to a track with your heart rate monitor. Start at a pace one minute per mile slower than your fastest predicted one mile time. Then, gradually increase the pace such that by the

fourth lap you are at your top one mile speed, and then give it all you've got for that last 200 meters. Your Max HR is the highest number registered on your heart rate monitor over those last 200 meters.

5. 800 Meter Format: Run 400 meters building to about the 95% level, then on the second 400 meters simulate a real race situation by trying to run as fast as you can. It actually helps me to have my fellow training partners with me during these track workouts, as they push me along.

Here's a print-out from one of my training friends:

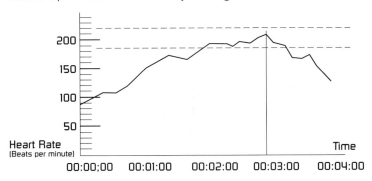

800 meter Max HR Test
Syd Winlock, 7/10/92, Hughes Stadium, Sacramento, CA

MAX HR TESTS: SWIMMING

1. Lap Test: Using your favorite stroke, swim 50 yards aggressively. Rest for two minutes. Using the time from your first 50 yards, add ten seconds to get your starting pace. Now, swim about six laps starting at this calculated pace. Each lap, try to decrease the lap time by five seconds until you can no longer increase your speed. Stop each 50 yards and look at your heart rate monitor. Your highest value during the test is equal to your Max HR.

MAX HR TESTS: CYCLING

1. Flat Terrain: Begin a "ladder" of 30 seconds intervals. At each 30 second "step," increase the speed of the bike by 1/2 mph (or 1 kph). There should be about 4-8 steps in the ladder, so your beginning speed needs to be about 2 mph slower than the rate of your fastest mid-distance, racing-speed.

2. Hilly Terrain: Find a long uphill or a series of hills, and after warming up, hit the bottom of the hill relatively fast. Work the hill extremely hard until your heart rate readings no longer rise and you approach exhaustion. This number is your Max HR.

CALCULATING YOUR RESTING HEART RATE

For some calculations of fitness and exercise intensity, it is helpful to determine your resting heart rate (Resting HR). The Resting HR is the number of beats for one minute when you are completely at rest. There are two ways of measuring Resting HR:

Morning Resting HR: Immediately after awakening and before you get out of bed, take your heart rate using your heart rate monitor or by counting the beats for 15 seconds and multiplying by four. I prefer to simply sleep with my heart rate monitor on and awake in the morning and read it first thing. Be warned, if your bladder is full in the morning, you didn't sleep well, or you're feeling stressed, you might have a slightly elevated Resting HR.

Evening Resting HR: Take a good book or magazine to bed and after 10-20 minutes in the prone position of quiet reading, take your heart rate. If you prefer, watch a calm television program for the 10-20 minute rest period while lying in the horizontal position.

Take both of these measurements for 7 days and average them. This average is your current Resting HR. This value is dependent on your lifestyle and a number of other factors such as quality of sleep, stress levels, and eating habits.

THE TRAINING HEART RATE CALCULATOR

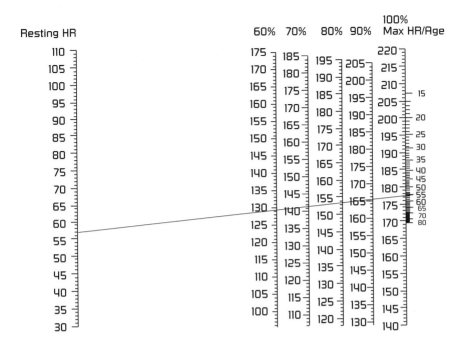

| Resting HR | | 60% | 70% | 80% | 90% | 100%
Max HR/Age | |

Training Heart Rate Calculator

The above chart is a nomograph, and it will make the math part of determining your maximum and target heart rates very simple. You don't see many nomographs nowadays, but they are ideal for our purposes because of their convenience. This particular nomograph is a state of the art model, designed with help from my friends Ned Frederick, Ph.D. Exercise Physiologist, and Larry Simpson, Mathematician, two exercise experts of the first order. They agree that calculating your target heart rates (THRs) is an extremely critical and highly necessary chore if one is to train smart. Simply wearing a heart rate monitor won't guarantee that you train smart unless you know how fast your heart should be beating during the various workouts you'll want to do.

NOTE: This calculator uses the Karvonen Formula to predict heart rate levels

As an example of how to use the Training Heart Rate Calculator, I've drawn a line across the nomograph to show how a 56 year-old, lifelong runner with a resting heart rate (RHR) of 52 bpm, would determine his or her maximum and target heart rates for several different effort levels. The left vertical axis of the Training Heart Rate Calculator is for RHR, and the right vertical axis is for maximum heart rate (MHR), whether age-predicted or actual. It's important to include RHR, since it reveals one's current level of fitness. In the example, the RHR gives our subject credit for having a fitness-induced RHR which is below normal. (The average RHRs for sedentary males and females are 72 and 84 bpm, respectively.)

You should already know how to determine your RHR: use your heart rate monitor to find your RHR several mornings in a row upon awakening, then average the figure. Find your RHR along the left vertical axis and mark it with a pen.

Unfortunately, determining your MHR is a little harder. Alert cardiologists have made us offer you three choices on the nomograph for marking your MHR:

CHOICE 1. For people who are absolutely sure of their actual MHR from treadmill stress testing, field tests, or from monitoring heart rate at the end of exhaustive workouts or races, use the numbers on the inside edge of the right vertical axis to find and note your exact MHR.

CHOICE 2. For adults who are just starting to exercise after living a sedentary lifestyle, find your age-adjusted MHR (as discussed in the preceding chapter) and match this predicted number to the numbers on the inside edge of the right vertical axis.

CHOICE 3. For exercisers who have stayed in shape most of their lives and who are known to be chronically fit, find your age among the numbers on the outside of the right vertical axis and use this as your mark-off point.

In my earlier example of a lifelong runner (he/she fits in the third category), by noting their RHR on the left vertical axis and their age on the outside of the right vertical axis, we can see that they would have a predicted MHR of 177 and predicted THRs for other intensity levels as noted. The method outlined in this example and in the third category was developed using the formula published by Dr. A. Hamid Hakki, et al, in the July 1983 issue of "Cardiovascular Reviews and Reports." The research of Dr. Hakki, a medical doctor at the William Likoff Cardiovascular Institute in Philadelphia, and similar efforts by Luger, et al, in Canada, has lead to the development of this MHR formula which is particularly accurate and well-suited for the chronically fit.

Still, for those in the second and third categories, you need to remember we're only guessing at your MHR based on statistical data. There could be a big difference in your actual MHR from the predictions in the nomograph, as much as ±30 bpm, especially for women and kids age 10–15. To be safe, those with special considerations should always have a physician determine your actual MHR. The other 80 or 90% of people out there will most likely fall inside the statistical bell curve and can safely rely on the chart.

Roy Benson, M.P.E., is a sports physiologist with a master's degree in physical education. Nicknamed "THE Runner's Coach," he is considered one of the best running coaches in the USA. His preference is for individualized coaching for all who are beginning a running program and for all runners who want to train to become their best. He can be reached by calling (404) 255-6234 or writing to Roy Benson, The Running Coach, 5600 Roswell Rd #355 Building North, Atlanta, GA 30342.

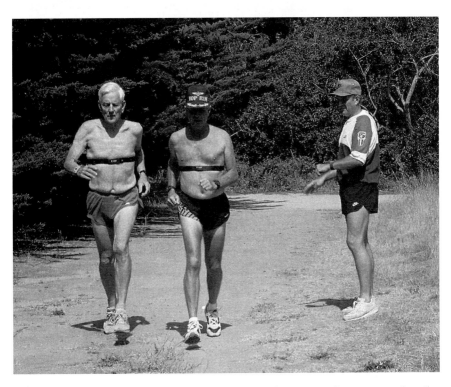

Roy Benson (far right) advising and encouraging several runners using the heart rate pace training method.

If we get right down to the mechanics of the thing, your heart is a sort of engine. You've got to check under your hood from time to time, watch your water levels, put in the right kind of fuel, and monitor its performance, just like you would for a car. Let the water levels drop or ignore its upkeep and sooner or later you're going to pay for it.

The Five Target

heart rate

zones

onsider your heart rate monitor to be a tachometer, which you can use to track your engine's progress, effort, and efficiency as you execute your training program. Just as you wouldn't want to red-line your car engine, you don't want to red-line your heart in its highest training zone very often.

There are five heart rate training zones in all. Training in one or all of these zones can play a part in your overall fitness or training program, depending on your individual goals. We use the term "zone" because target heart rates should not be thought of as a specific number of beats per minute. Rather, you need to think of training in the range within your target heart rate zone, say from 135 to 145 bpm. For example, the Moderate Activity zone ranges from 50% of your Max HR at its low end to 60% of your Max HR at its high end, so the zone then includes all of those heart rates within that range. Considering your heart rate's daily variations and fluctuations, it would be ridiculous to think that you should be shooting for one exact number day in and day out.

Finally, two things. First, when you figure out your training zone limits and want to enter them into your heart rate monitor, remember that monitors generally only take input in 5 bpm increments. So, if you are a dieter whose Moderate Activity zone extends from 80–96, you would set your lower training

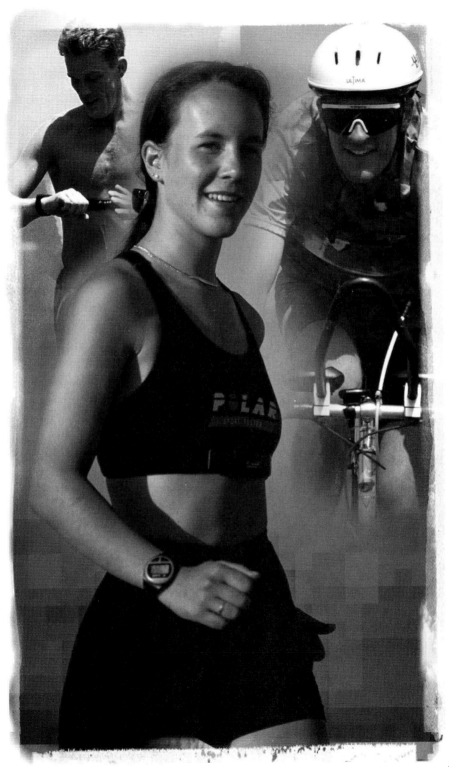

zone limit for 80 bpm, but you would have to round down (which is better than rounding up, if you are not very fit) from your actual upper limit of 96 bpm to 95 bpm for the monitor's setting. Second, this chapter may be long, but it is THE most important chapter in this book. Don't dare skip it. If you want, you can read it through section by section, but by all means read it to its end.

THE FIVE ZONES

There are five different heart rate training zones of five different levels of exercise intensity, each of which corresponds with various metabolic or respiratory transport mechanisms within your body. All of these zones can be tracked by your heart rate monitor; their values are as follows:

The Training Target Heart Zones

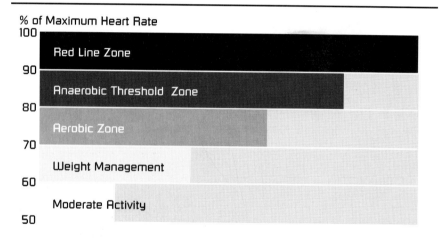

% of Maximum Heart Rate

- Red Line Zone
- Anaerobic Threshold Zone
- Aerobic Zone
- Weight Management
- Moderate Activity

THE MODERATE ACTIVITY ZONE: ....50 – 60% Max HR
THE WEIGHT MANAGEMENT ZONE: ..60 – 70% Max HR
THE AEROBIC ZONE: ....70 – 80% Max HR
THE ANAEROBIC THRESHOLD ZONE: 80 – 90% Max HR
THE RED-LINE ZONE: ....90 –100% Max HR

You will need to read on to learn how to figure out how much time you need to spend in each of these five target zones to achieve your personal fitness goals. Whether you are working out to lose weight or to reach peak performance levels, these training zones will be crucial to your success.

Each of the five target heart rates zones must be thoroughly understood for you to be able to design your own heart rate fitness program. To help you with this, included with the descriptions of each of the different zones is a chart that explains the zone and an example of a typical workout within that zone.

THE MODERATE ACTIVITY ZONE

This is probably one of the most important training zones and yet one of the least appreciated—especially by people in the "no pain, no gain" school of exercise. Many were taught that the major benefits of exercise were strength and speed. Although you are not streaking towards a four minute mile, training within the Moderate Activity zone will indeed increase your speed and strength. But even more, your body is going to be getting into shape by burning a higher blend of fat calories than carbohydrate calories for its fuel. This is the zone where "Long, Slow Distance" training comes into play.

Another reason the Moderate Activity zone has not received its due respect stems from the exercise scientist's term "fitness floor." Your Moderate Activity zone's heart rate range (50% to 60% of Max HR) happens to also be the initiation heart rate level for those who are beginning a training program and have been inactive, are in extremely poor condition, or who have to rehabilitate from a medical difficulty. It's also for those who are primarily interested in exercising for weight loss. In terms of exertion, training in the Moderate Activity zone should feel very relaxed and light. For further information see Chapter 10.

An example of the Moderate Activity zone in chart from is as follows:

Training Intensity Zone (% Max HR)	Maximum Heart Rate										
	150	155	160	165	170	175	180	185	190	195	200
Moderate Activity (50%-60%)	75 to 90	78 to 93	80 to 95	83 to 99	85 to 102	88 to 105	90 to 108	93 to 111	95 to 114	98 to 117	100 to 120

Finding your Moderate Activity zone is relatively easy. If you know your Max HR, multiply it by 50% for the low value and 60% for the high value of the range. Here's what the math formula looks like:

Moderate Activity Heart Rates:　Max HR_____ x .50 = ___ bpm
Max HR_____ x .60 = ___ bpm
Moderate Activity Zone: ____ to ____ bpm

Here's an example of a typical Moderate Activity zone workout program:

Walking: The 60 Minute Walk
This is a continuous 60 minute walk. If you need to slow down or stop to lower your heat rate, then do so. What's important is that you don't train below or above your Moderate Activity training zone. At first, make sure that you are on a flat course; a measured course such as a high school track is best, because you'll have a way to mark improvement. Program your heart rate monitor with the low and high heart rate limits for your Moderate Activity zone.

If you hear your heart rate monitor chirp, respond by increasing or decreasing your pace, as appropriate. Remember, if the alarm signals that you are outside your training zone, you need to respond immediately. The sound of that alarm is like a coach's voice telling you to go slower or faster. If you walk for longer than 60 minutes, it's all the better, since the longer the duration of Moderate Activity exercise, the more fat that burns!

WEIGHT MANAGEMENT ZONE

Training at this level will strengthen your heart and give it the opportunity to work at its optimum level.

The Weight Management zone ranges from 60% to 70% of your Max HR. It is also known as the "aerobic fitness threshold," because from this point forward, your body begins to reap the positive effects of aerobic exercise. This is the training zone that works your heart hard enough for it to get stronger and ready for a steady, pain-free, moderate pace.

Here's how to determine your Weight Management zone. If you know your Max HR, multiply it by 60% for the low value and 70% for the high value. Here's what the math formula looks like:

Weight Management Rates: Max HR_____ x .60 = ___ bpm
Max HR_____ x .70 = ___ bpm
Weight Management Zone : ____ to ____ bpm

An example of this range in chart form is as follows:

Training Intensity Zone (% Max HR)	*Weight Management Zone*										
	150	155	160	165	170	175	180	185	190	195	200
Weight Management (60%-70%)	90 to 105	93 to 109	96 to 112	99 to 116	102 to 119	105 to 123	108 to 126	111 to 130	114 to 133	117 to 137	120 to 140

An example of a typical Weight Management zone workout program, if you cycle, would be as follows:

Cycling: Training Ride
Begin with an easy five minute warm-up; try "spinning," pedalling lightly and quickly in a low gear as you work through those beginning few minutes. This should put your heart rate near your Weight Management training zone. Fix on a certain speed if you have a cyclometer or just sense an even pace and try and hold this at the top end of your Weight Management zone for five minutes. Then slow down until you are at the lowest value for this zone and ride for five more minutes. This is an example of a criss-cross workout during

which you vary the heart rate intensity and speed for alternating intervals of rest and training, and you can repeat the stages as many times as you wish. For maximum Weight Management zone benefits, I recommend spending 30–60 minutes on this workout.

Cycling: Recovery Ride

This is a great ride if you're coming off a hard workout the day before. It's a steady-state ride designed to facilitate recovery from a hard training ride or race within the prior 24–48 hours, while still giving you other benefits of working out. The distance of the ride should be relatively short and the duration no longer than 60 minutes. Just program your heart rate monitor with the lower (60% Max HR) and upper limits (70% Max HR) of your training zone, and use your monitor to stay within them.

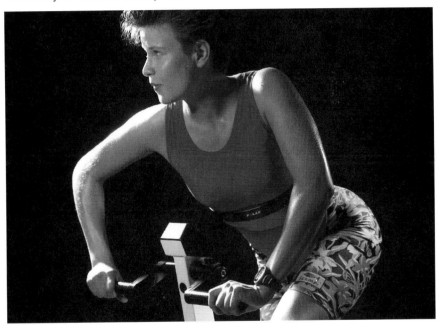

The Aerobic Zone makes you feel the workout, your heart rate, and the training effects.

THE AEROBIC ZONE

Training within the aerobic zone benefits not only your heart, but also your "respiratory" or breathing system (the other half of the "cardio-respiratory" equation). Training your respiratory system is what increases your endurance. When training within this range, you enhance your aerobic power, the ability to transport oxygen to and carbon dioxide away from the sport-specific muscles. The aerobic zone is the standard training zone which for years has been called "the target heart rate zone," but which in fact should have been called the "aerobic target heart rate zone," since it is but one of the five target heart rate zones.

At 70%–80% of your Max HR, your workout times and effort levels will both begin to drop after several weeks. If, for example, you are now able to jog a mile within this heart rate range in ten minutes, within a few weeks you should be able to jog that same distance in less time in the same aerobic target zone. This improvement is called "the training effect."

So, if you are exercising to increase your aerobic capacity, this is your primary training zone. If you were asked to describe the intensity of this level you would say that it was "somewhat hard," and indeed that is what you will feel. At this heart rate intensity you are going to feel some of the discomforts of the exercise regimen. It is not a painful training zone, like the red-line, but it is one that will get you breathing strongly, working hard, and feeling the exertions of your body.

To determine this aerobic heart rate zone, if you know your Max HR, multiply your Max HR by 70% for the low value and 80% for the high value. Here's what the math formula looks like:

Aerobic Heart Rates: Max HR_____ x .70 = ___ bpm
                        Max HR_____ x .80 = ___ bpm
                        Aerobic Zone : ____ to ____ bpm

An example of the aerobic target heart rate range in chart form is as follows:

Training Intensity Zone (% Max HR)	Maximum Heart Rate										
	150	155	160	165	170	175	180	185	190	195	200
Aerobic (70%-80%)	105 to 120	109 to 124	112 to 128	116 to 132	119 to 136	123 to 140	126 to 144	130 to 148	133 to 152	137 to 156	140 to 160

The benefits of exercising in the aerobic heart rate zone are enormous. Sure, you burn a higher percentage of carbohydrates than fats as your fuel, but you also strengthen both your heart and your lungs by demanding higher workloads. If you want to get fitter, faster, and stronger, train in the aerobic heart rate zone.

Here's an example of an aerobic zone training swim:
Swimming: Over-distance Swim
This is a perfect Sunday morning, over-distance training workout at slower than race pace. Set the limits on your wrist monitor to 70% (low threshold) and 80% (high threshold of your Max HR). This should be an approximately 30 minute, relaxed, steady swim, in a pool or open, fresh water.* With time, you should be able to learn this pace so well that you'll never hear the limit alarm sound.

THE ANAEROBIC THRESHOLD ZONE

At this level you are training near the point where aerobic training crosses over and becomes anaerobic training. At some point within this zone, from 80% to 90% of your Max HR, you will be training at or near your anaerobic threshold. When training within this range, the primary benefit is to increase your body's ability to metabolize lactic acid, allowing you to train harder before crossing over into the pain of lactate accumulation and oxygen debt.

If you were asked to describe the intensity of this level you would say that it was "hard." You are going to feel the pain that comes with training hard— tired muscles, heavy breathing, and fatigue. If you keep with it though, in return the training effect will occur, and you will be able to sustain more work over longer amounts of time at lower heart rate levels.

To calculate your personal anaerobic training zone, multiply your Max HR by 80% for the low value and 90% for the high value. Here's what the math formula looks like:

Anaerobic Threshold Heart Rates: Max HR_____ x .80 = ___ bpm

Max HR_____ x .90 = ___ bpm

Anaerobic Zone : ____ to ____ bpm

An example of the anaerobic target heart rate range in chart form is as follows:

Training Intensity Zone (% Max HR)	Maximum Heart Rate										
	150	155	160	165	170	175	180	185	190	195	200
Anaerobic (80%-90%)	120 to 135	124 to 140	128 to 144	132 to 149	136 to 153	140 to 158	144 to 162	148 to 167	152 to 171	156 to 176	160 to 180

Note: While water resistant heart rate monitors are guaranteed not to be damaged by water, they are not guaranteed to function in all types of water. For example, in all salt water and some chemically-treated pool situations, the high conductivity of the water will cause your transmitter's signal to scatter and not reach your monitor. In short, swimming in the ocean with your heart rate monitor is not a fruitful activity.

The benefits of exercising in the anaerobic threshold heart rate zone are primarily for those who are interested in high performance training. If you just want to be fit, you probably don't need to spend much time (if any) within this zone. If, however, your goal is to beat the clock or a fellow training partner, you need to spend several workouts a week within this zone.

Here's an example of a typical anaerobic threshold zone workout program for a runner preparing for a race, by Owen Anderson, editor and publisher of "Running Research News"*:

<u>Running: The 10k Race Pace—"Lactate Threshold Criss-Cross"</u>

This workout is designed to raise your anaerobic threshold (AT) heart rate level. Your 10k race pace is slightly higher than your AT level, so training at this pace will help lift your AT heart rate higher.

*"Running Research News" is a bimonthly newsletter which provides endurance athletes with important new information about training, sports nutrition, and sports medicine. Famed running coach Arthur Lydiard says, " 'Running Research News' is outstanding. It does the best job of all the running publications at interpreting scientific information and providing practical pointers for endurance athletes." Subscriptions to "Running Research News" are $17 per year. Please call 1-800-333-FEET or write to RRN, P.O. Box 27041, Lansing, MI 48909 for more information.

I first set the heart rate monitor's upper alarm at a heart rate typical of my 10k races and the lower alarm at 12 beats per minute below the upper alarm, in my case, the higher alarm sounds at 180 beats per minute and the lower at 170. [Editor's Note: Since the majority of heart rate monitors' training zone

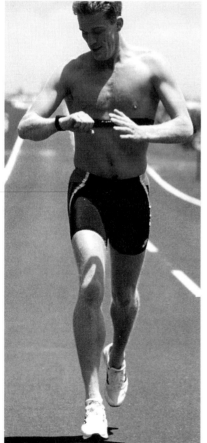

limits can only be set in 5 bpm increments, instead of a 12 bpm training zone range, you will likely set a range of 10 or 15 bpm and work from there accordingly.]

After I warm up by jogging easily for about ten minutes, I increase my running pace so that the lower alarm stops sounding, and I then run fairly easily at a heart rate of 172-175 for a few minutes. After that I accelerate gradually until the higher alarm goes off, at which point I slowly decrease my speed until the lower alarm begins beeping again. The rest of the workout consists of moving back and forth between these upper and lower limits (I often spend about two minutes on each ascent or descent).

I call this workout the "lactate threshold (LT) criss-cross," because a runner's actual lactate threshold running

During a criss-cross running session, the alarms of your heart rate monitor will beep when you are above or below your pre-set zones.

speed usually corresponds with a heart rate within this 12-beat heart rate zone. The workout activates the various types of leg muscle cells—slow twitch, fast twitch A, and fast twitch B—and has a very positive impact on lactate threshold and VO2 max (maximal aerobic capacity).

The criss-cross is a great specific workout, too, because it forces runners to develop the appropriate nerve-muscle coordination patterns necessary for excellent 10k racing.

Although the LT criss-cross is an intense workout, it's also very relaxing. For one thing, you don't have to worry about your actual running speed; keeping your heart rate within the 12-beat zone will ensure that you get a great workout. As you do the criss-cross, you can relax and concentrate totally on good form and pace adjustment—the heart rate monitor's alarms will do everything else.

Beginning runners should shoot for 6–8 minutes within the criss-cross zone for their first workout, but experienced runners often run continuously for about 20–25 minutes per session. A nice cool-down jog always follows the criss-cross, which can be easily carried out in your favorite running location. One final point: for the upper heart rate limit, don't use 10k heart rates from races run under extreme conditions, such as high heat, humidity, or wind, unless almost all your running is done in those situations.

THE RED-LINE ZONE

This is the highest intensity training. You should only train at this level if you are extremely fit. While you are in the red-line, you will have crossed over the anaerobic threshold, and you will be operating in oxygen debt, meaning that your muscles will be using more oxygen than your body can provide. That's ok, because if you will recall, skeletal muscles operate under the "work now, pay later" principle.

By definition, the red-line training zone is 90–100% of your Max HR. That means stomping your foot on the throttle and going as fast as you can for brief periods of time. You are going to be training the metabolic pathways of your fast twitch muscles, not your endurance pathways or enzymes. This is extremely difficult training and should only be used by those who are aspiring to their highest levels.

If you were asked to describe what it feels like to train within the red-line zone, the response would be colorful, full of expletives, and entirely unprintable. The "rigs" or rigor mortis, as athletes describe it, start to set in at this level. You will be breathing in short breaths at the highest frequency possible. You will feel like you can't breathe enough oxygen and that your heart is working so hard that it wants to jump out of your chest. In other words, this is training at the max of the max.

If you know your Max HR, multiply it by 90% for the low value and 100% for the high value of your red-line range. The high value will be the highest number your have ever seen on your Heart rate monitor.

Here's what the math formula looks like:

Red-line Heart Rates: Max HR_____ x . 90 = ___ bpm
Max HR_____ x 1.00 = ___ bpm
Red-line Zone : ____ to ____ bpm

An example of the red-line target heart rate range in chart form is as follows:

Training Intensity Zone (% Max HR)	*Maximum Heart Rate*										
	150	155	160	165	170	175	180	185	190	195	200
Red Line (90%-100%)	135 to 150	140 to 155	144 to 160	149 to 165	153 to 170	158 to 175	162 to 180	167 to 185	171 to 190	176 to 195	180 to 200

The red-line target heart rate zone is a very special and revered place. It is not an area of training that one should enter frequently or without a great deal of appreciation and respect. If you spend too much time in this "pain and gain" zone you put a lot on the line, because it is definitely a high risk zone. This is the area of training that frequently leads to injuries from overuse problems. The red-line zone is not for the faint of heart, but rather for those who have trained extensively, have a working knowledge of the principles of high performance training, and want to get a lot faster—quickly.

An example of a typical red-line heart zone workout program, if you were a cross-country skier would be as follows:

Cross-Country Skiing: The 5k Race Pace
You can maintain your AT threshold level heart rate for just less than one hour. To train above the AT level, break the workout into multiple 5k intervals and then train at or just below your 5k racing pace. Your 5k racing pace is equivalent to training at 5% to 10% below your Max HR. If you want to ski fast, you need to train fast.

REVIEW: YOUR FIVE HEART RATE TRAINING ZONES IN PERSPECTIVE

You've made it! You now know about the five target heart rate zones and will soon (if you haven't already) figure them out for yourself. You MUST take the time to do this. The next step will be to put your training zone information together into a heart rate monitor fitness program, and this will be discussed further in the following chapters. For now, realize that getting a healthier heart, losing some pounds, or increasing your aerobic ability requires training at specific, monitored levels. Once you understand the dynamics of these levels, you'll be able to streamline your training program to get to where you're going safely and efficiently and in less time.

To assist you in putting together all the information I've thrown at you, I've included the following review chart on the next page.

Heart Rate Zone	*The five training heart rates - review*					
	%Max HR	%Max VO2	Workout duration	System Trained	Max Pace	Term for zone
Moderate Activity	50% - 60%	Up to 50%	60+ min.	Metabolic Fuel Burning	Walking/ Striding	Easy Pace
Weight Management	60% - 70%	50% - 60%	30+ min.	Cardio-respiratory	Marathon	Base Work
Aerobic	70% - 80%	60% - 75%	8-30 min.	Aerobic	10 K	Long
Anaerobic	80% - 90%	75% - 85%	5-8 min.	Lactate Clearance	3 k - 5 k	Tempo
Red-Line	90% - 100%	85% - 100%	1-5 min.	Anaerobic	800 meters - 1500 meters	Short

Some of my friends have complained that there's too much math in this book. I empathize. But, to use a heart rate monitor effectively, you are going to have to know the values for your individual heart rates. You are going to need to post them somewhere so when you say, "this is an aerobic workout," you can program your heart rate monitor with your individual aerobic training zone. I have designed the following personal chart for you to use. Photocopy it and then post it so you are aware of your own individual zones.

A healthy heart is worth spending a little time with a calculator and a piece of paper, don't you think?

THE FIVE TRAINING HEART RATE ZONES

Date:

Your Name:

		Low HR	High HR
1.	MODERATE ACTIVITY ZONE: 50%-60% Max HR	_____ bpm to	_____ bpm
2.	WEIGHT MANAGEMENT ZONE: 60%-70% Max HR	_____ bpm to	_____ bpm
3.	AEROBIC ZONE: 70%-80% Max HR	_____ bpm to	_____ bpm
4.	ANAEROBIC THRESHOLD ZONE: 80%-90% Max HR	_____ bpm to	_____ bpm
5.	RED-LINE ZONE: 90%-100% Max HR	_____ bpm to	_____ bpm

From the Heart Rate Monitor Book, by Sally Edwards. Permission granted to reproduce and post.

GUESSTIMATING YOUR ANAEROBIC THRESHOLD

In training the endurance athlete, one goal I strive to attain is to teach my clients to train effectively. The best way I have found to do so is by varying the intensity of each training session in order to stress different energy systems and evoke appropriate physiological adaptations from each type of training. In short, I feel it is essential to train smarter by training hard when the plan calls for hard effort and to train easily when the plan calls for easy effort. I've found that it's the hard, high intensity training that poses the most significant challenge to athletes and brings up the most questions, such as:

"What heart rate should I use for interval training?"
"How do I know when I'm at my anaerobic threshold?"
"What pace should I use for improving my anaerobic threshold?"

These questions are quite valid and are worthy of some answers.

Since most of us do not have access to high tech physiology labs, we need to rely on other means to "guesstimate" our training intensity levels. I've found that there are three variables we can use to determine this intensity. These three variables are (1) actual heart rate; (2) subjective feeling or

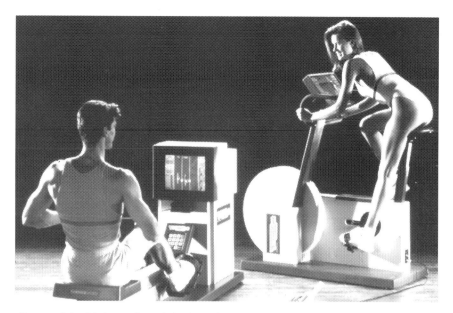

Some of the high quality original equipment manufacturers have incorporated the heart rate measurement technology into their own fitness machines.

perceived exertion; and (3) actual pace or time per set distance. It is very useful for the athlete to develop an ability to make a relationship between the three distinct, yet interdependent, variables associated with training intensity levels.

Intervals, hills, speed work, time-trials, race pace, fartlek, repeats—all these terms may be used to describe high intensity training that is designed to increase the body's ability to sustain the highest speed possible for race distances. If you measure your heart rate, you will find that this training takes place at between 80-95% of your maximum heart rate. Your subjective feelings, rated on a scale of 1 to 10 (with 10 as exhaustion), would rank between a 7 and 9. Speed, in terms of miles per hour, minutes per mile, minutes per kilometer, or meters per second, would vary depending upon the individual, fitness level, biomechanical efficiency, etc. I've found that the athlete can use all of these parameters to fine-tune efficiency, anaerobic threshold, and the ability to sustain top race speed appropriate for a given race distance, and I suggest that athletes perform the following test to achieve the goal of maximally effective training:

THE TEST: ANAEROBIC THRESHOLD TEST

Purpose: To test the Anaerobic Threshold and use and adjust the level of intensity in training.

Equipment: A reliable heart rate monitor (Polar is the best I've used); a stop watch; and a performance log where you can record date, distance, time, average heart rate during the effort, and subjective feeling.

Test Protocol:

1) Choose a specific location that will be reliable and repeatable. This could be a favorite stretch of road, a running track, your local swimming pool, etc. The distances can vary for each athlete, but once you settle on a distance, stick with that same exact course and distance for each test you perform over the months. It's ideal if you can mark your courses with 1 kilometer markings. Choose a distance that takes you about 15-30 minutes to complete, for example, for running, 5 k, for cycling, 20 k, and for swimming, 1000 meters.

2) Warm up for 15 minutes at low to medium intensity before starting the test.

3) Perform the test distance at a pace that is the fastest you feel you can sustain at a steady effort with no loss of speed. Heart rate should stabilize in about five minutes. Start your timer as you begin the test and record your time for the distance when you finish. The heart rate you achieved and sustained is your anaerobic threshold heart rate. Also, record your subjective feeling of difficulty you had during the test.

4) Do a 15 minute cool-down and some stretching after the workout is over.

Testing Frequency: Do this test once each month for each sport in which you are competing. If you are a triathlete, do the test for cycling the first week, running the next, and swimming the third week. It is important to substitute this test in place of a scheduled interval, hill interval, or race pace workout.

Special Considerations: After each test, take some time to look over the relationship between your heart rate, subjective feeling, and pace per km which you sustained during the test. Use these three variables to fine-tune your anaerobic threshold, heart rate, and pace. Then for the coming four weeks, do your intervals, hill intervals, and race pace workouts at between 1–10 heartbeats per minute (bpm) lower than your anaerobic threshold bpm. You'll probably adjust this after next month's test. Eventually, you'll fine-tune these three variables so that if you need to, you'll be able to rely on subjective feeling and pace per km with the same credibility as heart rate.

Rob Sleamaker, M.S., is a sports physiologist and author of SERIOUS Training For SERIOUS Athletes (Human Kinetics Publishers, 1-800-747-4457). He is the creator of the SportsAdvantage™ Personalized Training System, a unique systematic training program for endurance athletes and multi-sport fitness enthusiasts. Rob also invented the Vasa Swim Trainer, an exercise machine used by world-class swimmers and triathletes. Rob conducts SportsAdvantage™ multi-sport clinics and seminars the world over. For information about these products and services, call 1-802-660-9660.

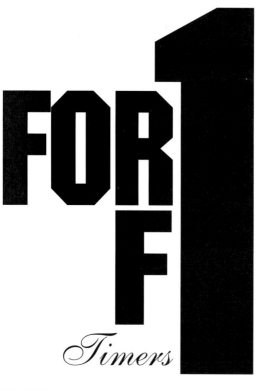

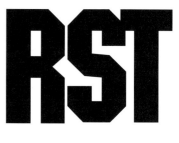

CHAPTER SEVEN

Dick McKenzie, a retired 64 year-old living in Alabama, purchased a heart rate monitor over a year ago. He carefully read the manual and was soon able to program his training zones into his wrist monitor. In principal he was ready. The problem was, in practice he didn't know what to do next.

here's a lot more to using a heart rate monitor than just knowing how to program it. This chapter will give you a step-by-step, easy to follow guide on how to use your heart rate monitor after you have become friends with it.

If you follow each step carefully, you won't have to do what Dick had to do, call me and get a personal lesson.

STEP #1:

<u>Calculate each of your five target heart rate zones.</u>

Refer back to chapter six where you were shown how to complete all of the calculations for your five target zones: the moderate activity zone, the weight management zone, the aerobic zone, the anaerobic zone, and the red-line zone.

STEP #2:

<u>Write down your goals.</u>

You have committed to using a heart rate monitor because you want to accomplish something. What is it that you want? Answer the question: Why am I exercising or thinking about starting a program? You probably will have more than one goal, so list them on the next page:

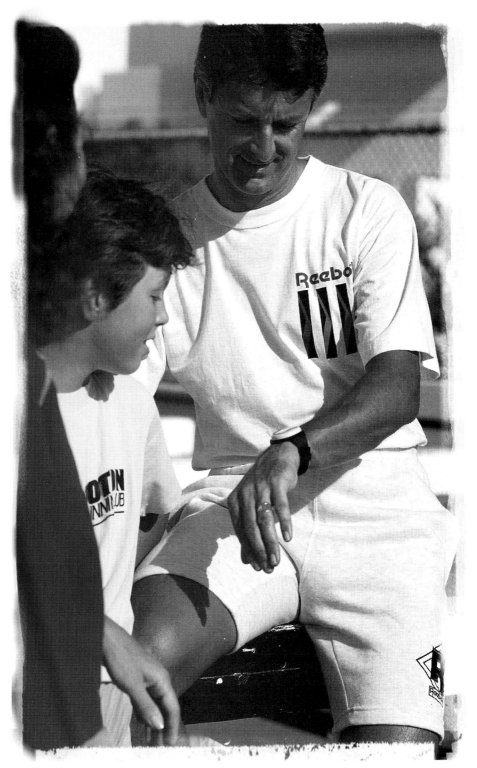

LIST OF GOALS

	Goal to Accomplish	Amount	Date
1.			
2.			
3.			
4.			
5.			

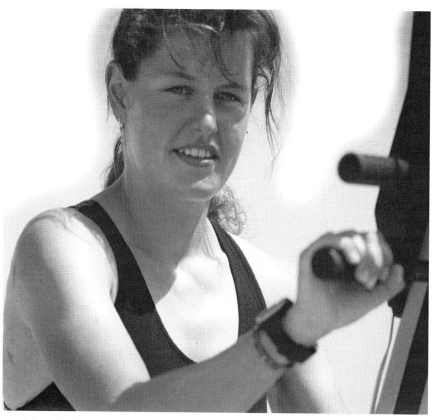

Most individuals exercise not because they love to, but because they want something out of it: a slimmer figure, the ability to walk up a flight of stairs without huffing and puffing, maybe even to enhance recovery from a heart attack, or improve their golf game. You must be specific here and list your exact goals; just putting down "to lose some weight" is not specific enough. If you wish to lose weight, how much do you want to lose? By when? Be quantitative with all of your goals and remember that setting and meeting goal dates can be more important than the contents of the goals themselves!

STEP #3:

Write down a training plan.

This doesn't take a coach or an exercise physiologist. It's just a daily planner for your workouts, and it looks like this:

The Plan					The Log					NRZ Setting Summary
Day/Date	Sport	Time/Dist	High	Low	Sport	Time/Dist	Below	In	Above	Notes & Comments
M										☺☺☺ Resting HR: WR
T										☺☺☺ Resting HR: WR
W										☺☺☺ Resting HR: WR
T										☺☺☺ Resting HR: WR
F										☺☺☺ Resting HR: WR
S										☺☺☺ Resting HR: WR
S										☺☺☺ Resting HR: WR

Plan Summary — Total # Workouts: **Log Summary** — Total # Workouts: **Weekly goals accomplished** ☺ ☹

Total Time: HR Zone Time Total: Fixed   Total Time: HR Zone Time Total: Fixed   Comments:

AT: Aerobic   Healthy   Fat   AT: Aerobic   Healthy   Fat

For most first-timers, the three low intensity target zone types are the most important: the moderate activity zone, the weight management zone, and the aerobic zone. Under the column headed "target zone type," fill in which of these you want to accomplish on which days. Then fill in your target heart rates that correspond with each of these zones and describe what type of activities you are going to do to attain your goals for that day. Include all the details you can think of, i.e., warm-ups, location, and specific main workout.

Here are five simple rules for filling out your training plan:

1) Schedule a minimum of three to four workouts per week.
2) Make sure that all workouts are within the target ranges.
3) Variety is important. Get into cross-training by planning walking one day, aerobics another, and cycling on a third. It's also fine to repeat activities as you see fit.
4) At least two workouts should be of the same target training zone type as your priority goal, i.e., moderate activity or weight management zones for weight loss.
5) Set a minimum of 15 minutes and maximum of 30-60 minutes for each workout in

STEP #4:

Set your heart rate monitor.

Put on your heart rate monitor. Program your training limits and the time/duration of the workout. If you have a recovery rate function, program somewhere between one and four minutes for a recovery period. Read chapter 8, "How To Train with Your Heart Rate Monitor," for more in-depth advice.

STEP #5:

Complete the plan for that day.

The road to fitness hell is paved with good intentions. Planning something is always easier than doing it. The benefits of using a heart rate monitored program can only be realized if you execute the workouts.

STEP #6:

Record your training session achievements.

We have provided you with a sample of a useful combination of a planning guide and a workout log on the previous page. You can photocopy it or order one of your own called the Heart Rate Monitor Logbook from your local dealer or FLEET FEET SPORTS (send a check or money order to 2408 "J" Street, Sacramento, CA 95816 for $10, shipping and handling included). The point of this journal is that it helps you plan your heart rate monitor program in advance and then allows you to log in your accomplishments into the same book for easy comparison.

Let's take you through Dick McKenzie's experience. After we met for thirty minutes, Dick was able to write down his goals and design his exercise plan. Here are his goals and his dreams:

GOAL	CURRENT AMOUNT	GOAL AMOUNT	DUE DATE
1. lose 5lbs.	185 lbs.	180 lbs.	4 wks.
2. lower resting HR by 5 bpm	65 bpm	60 bpm	5 wks.
3. improve my aerobic capacity	Walk 1 mile in 15 min. 130 bpm	Walk 1 mile in 14 min 130 bpm	4 wks.
4. to run in my first 5k race	have never done before	to do it!	8 wks.

To accomplish these goals, Dick needed to write down his weekly workouts for eight weeks. He wrote his planned program in his Planner Log, then he logged his daily accomplishments. This is a sample of what one week looked like:

Day/Date	The Plan — Sports	Time/Dist.	HRZ Setting — High	Low	The Log — Sports	Time/Dist.	HRZ Setting Summary — Below	In	Above	Notes & Comments
M 63/83	WALK	1 mile	130	110	Walk	1 mile	2 min	12 min	1 min	Resting HR ___ Wt. ___ Feel good - more sleep.
T 63/83	WALK	1 mile	130	110	Walk	1 mile	4 min	10 min	1 min	Resting HR ___ Wt. ___ A little sluggish today - lake was beautiful!
W 63/83	walk	1 mile	130	110						Resting HR ___ Wt. ___ meetings & travel
T 63/87	walk	1 mile	120	110	walk	1 mile	1 min	12 min	2 min	Resting HR ___ Wt. ___ feel great! 14 min mile!
F 63/83	Walk	"	"	"	"	"	3 min	10 min	2 min	Resting HR ___ Wt. ___ Nice & easy today great weather
S 63/83	"	"	"	"	"	"	2	10	2	Resting HR ___ Wt. ___ Resting heart rate dropped to 62!
S 63/83	"	"	"	"	Tennis /					Resting HR ___ Wt. ___ 110-140 bpm lot of fun. I about 75 min.

Plan Summary
Total Time: 1:45   AT: /   Aerobic: /
Total # Workouts: 7
HR Zone Time Totals: Red /   Healthy: 1:45   Fat: /

Log Summary
Total Time: 2   AT: /   Aerobic: 20
Total # Workouts: 6
HR Zone Time Totals: Red /   Healthy: 1:30   Fat: 10

Weekly goals accomplished ☺☺
Comments: feeling healthier look out 5K - I'm ready!

Let's say Dick really wanted to start a step aerobic program. How would he use his heart rate monitor for this? Simple. He would use the same six steps listed before, but would tailor them for a step aerobic format: how many times per week he was taking the class, what his goals were, and which of his five target heart rate zones were aligned with those goals. This process is the same for every activity, from tennis to snowshoeing.

With that, Dick was off and running, and you can be, too. Don't let anything hold you back—I'm right here behind you.

MULTI-SPORT MAXIMUM HEART RATE DIFFERENCES

When I first started using a heart rate monitor, I used the formulas to determine my maximum heart rate and training zone percentages, and I found that my actual norms were always outside the heart rate zones. My heart rate was always too high for the formulas. Also, even though I started with a higher heart rate than predicted when training, it would always quickly rise still higher, but then I could maintain that same heart rate at the same pace for longer than my training partners. Their heart rates would drift upwards with time, while we trained at the same pace, and my heart rate would have little to no upward drift. The bottom line is that even though most people (80%) are supposed to be able to use heart rate formulas accurately, there are still a good number of us who, for health and safety reasons, really have to figure things out on our own.

At the 1991 Hawaii Ironman Triathlon, I competed with a Polar Vantage XL heart rate monitor and set my racing heart rate values for 145-150 bpm for the 112 mile bike leg and at 155-160 bpm for the 26.2 mile marathon. I wouldn't have finished the race, the most difficult in my life, without a heart rate monitor. Actually, I wouldn't race at any distance without one.

I was curious as to whether my Max HR was the same in all three of my triathlon sports. To determine my Max HR in running, I did three one mile repeats, with the first at about 80% of Max HR, the second at 90% Max HR, and the third mile I go all out and hammer it. I determined my running Max HR to be 201 bpm, and at the age of 33 years, the age-adjusted formulas predict it to be 187 bpm. This is a 14 bpm error, too great for any serious athlete's purposes.

Still, I have found on the bike that the formula is pretty accurate. I took a ten mile time trial, and each mile I shifted into a harder gear until I maxed out at 186 bpm.

The Max HR protocol that I follow for swimming is as follows. First I do a 500 yard warm-up. Then I do a 5 x 50 yards main set, reducing the rest time by five seconds with each departure, down to a ten second rest. Simultaneously, I increase the split pace from 47 seconds to 35 seconds. This routine allowed me to find out that my maximum heart rate for swimming is 175 bpm!

I can't tell you why there is such a difference in my Max HR among swimming (175 bpm), running (201 bpm), and cycling (186 bpm)—I just know that for me it exists. I think it is essential that all multi-sport athletes take a Max HR test in each of their specific sports and then calculate their training percentages based on each sport's Max HR.

One of my favorite and almost daily workout activities is to play a game called "guessing my heart rate." I say to myself, "My heart rate right now is between 145-150 (I always use a range)." I win if I am within five beats of what my heart rate monitor says, and at this point, I am right about 95% of the time. This game is also a way for me to hone my perception of perceived effort and real effort. I now can race and be within 2-3 bpm of my heart rate goal without having to look at my heart rate monitor. This training has helped me tremendously when I race, because now I can keep to my heart rate-based race strategy and not someone else's. It has taken me almost two years to develop what I call my "ninth sense," the ability to perceive and know my heart rate through the entire range from rest to Max HR, and I have my heart rate monitor to thank for it.

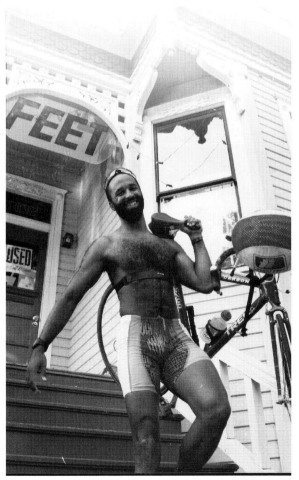

Syd Winlock is the Senior Vice-President of FLEET FEET, Incorporated, an international franchisor of sports retail stores. He is author Sally Edwards' primary training partner, and together they have developed a great deal of the information in The Heart Rate Monitor Book by practical use of heart rate monitors in their daily training. Syd finished the 1991 Ironman in 13 hours.

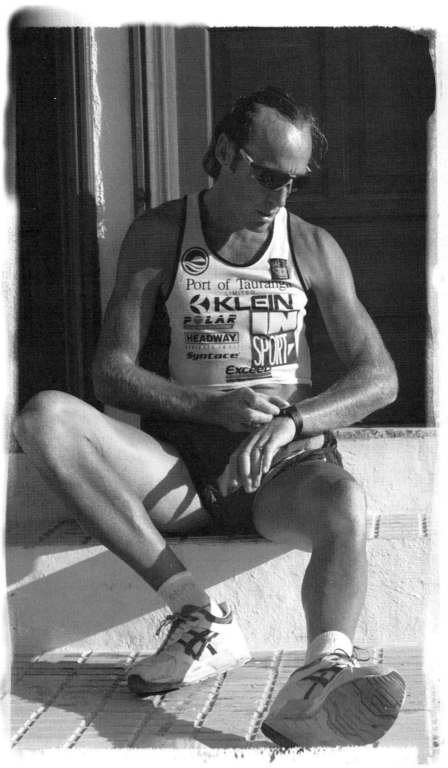

How

to train with a heart

rate

My legs were spinning as I watched the display on my heart rate monitor climb to 175 beats per minute and my cyclometer read-out jump to 21 mph. I could feel my breath start to burn my chest and the blood pounding in my temples. "My heart," I thought, "must think I'm crazy." Of course my lungs, legs, back, knees, and feet had found that out long ago. I have felt them saying, "This hurts, STOP IT!!!" during the longest of my endurance races. Still, over the past 25 years of racing, they've come to accept my stubbornness and stamina.

monitor

ut after all those years of training, here was this new high tech toy, this heart rate monitor, telling me that I was maxing out. Maxing out? Red-lining! Me? My heart rate continued to race at 175 bpm, and I pushed on. Mind over body, I thought. Damn the torpedoes.

180 bpm came and went. 182 bpm. My hands tingled. 185 bpm. Ouch. Head down, knees pumping, I fought to disprove what my heart rate monitor was telling me, "You're going too hard."

To make a long story short, it didn't take long for me to burn out—30 seconds, to be exact. I spent the rest of the ride at a steady pace of 160 bpm, licking my wounds and thinking that maybe, just maybe, my heart rate monitor was my friend, not my competition.

It's not a matter of listening to an electronic device strapped to your wrist. It's about listening to your heart and linking your mind with your body. Once you learn to monitor and understand your body, you'll be on your way to an efficient, effective training program.

SETTING UP YOUR HEART RATE MONITOR
BEFORE YOUR WORKOUT

From the simplest to the most complex heart rate monitor models, there are some basic concepts and techniques you need to learn in order to make the most of a heart rate monitor and of your workout.

If your unit displays nothing but your heart rate, then jot down your workout plan in advance, including: one of your five training zones, your maximum heart rate (Max HR), and the time period you would like to spend within the training zone. Then as you train, periodically check the wrist monitor and make a mental note of the session. Note your beginning heart rate, your final heart rate and your two-minute recovery rate. Also note your highs and lows within specific training zones (TZ). A great workout is one in which your written plan matches your actual performance.

The best place to write down your exercise information is in your training log or planner. Because of the specific needs and features of heart rate monitor training programs, we have designed a specific log for you to record your training data (see the preceding chapter for more details). Ideally, you'll get better and better at matching your performance to your training plan.

Mid-priced heart rate monitors will provide you with a number of helpful features. Most of these models provide some programmability, such as the ability to set the limits of your training zone, the two heart rate levels that you wish to train within. At your Weight Management intensity, the upper end of your training zone would be at 70% of your Max HR, say 135 bpm. If you train too hard and your heart rate rises above this value, an alarm will sound with each heart beat to signal that you need to decrease your training intensity. This can be particularly helpful for those of you who have a tendency to train too hard during your workouts. Similarly, if you aren't training hard enough and your heart rate drops to the lower TZ limit, the alarm will signal that you need to pick up your effort.

Top of the line heart rate monitors offer an amazing range of features. They can store a continuous heart rate for over 33 hours in eight separate files. If you want to store eight different workouts, you can do so before you download the information into a computer or manually record it in your log book. If you cross train, this feature really comes in handy—you can store multiple workouts in different files and analyze the information at your leisure. To go along with these high-end monitors, you can purchase a computer interface package and software that performs an in-depth analysis of your workout information. The software is available for either Macintosh or IBM PC systems, and using it is surprisingly easy. Once you place the wrist monitor on the interface unit, all you do is push a button on the wrist monitor, and bingo, your entire heart rate workout is there on your personal computer screen.

Once you have downloaded the data, you can graph and print out your entire workout for your records. The software will also analyze your individual aerobic and anaerobic thresholds (upper and lower Max HR percentages, for example) and the percentage of time you are training below, within, or above those levels. It also calculates your average heart rate—one of my favorite features.

For serious athletes, there has never been a better personal source of training data.

THE WORKOUT: USING YOUR HEART RATE MONITOR

Let's go through a workout and look at how you can use your heart rate monitor data collector to give you critical training information.

First, set up the parameters of the workout. If you've got a monitor with the capability, program how many minutes you want for a warm-up and then how many minutes you want for a cool-down period. The heart rate monitor beeper will signal the duration of these sessions. Let's say you want 10% of your 60 minute workout to be warm-up and 10% to be cool-down. You would then program a 6 minute warm-up and a 6 minute cool-down period. This leaves you with a 48 minute training set. If your monitor doesn't have these capabilities, use a wrist watch or stopwatch to time your warm-up, training set, and cool-down; these steps are too important to not measure accurately.

Next, enter the target heart rate zone limits for your workout. If you are training in your aerobic training zone and your Max HR measures 175 bpm, then your TZ consists of the lower 123 bpm (rounded to 125 bpm) limit and the upper 145 bpm limit.

Now look at your workout. You can either run, ride, ski, etc., a steady pace or you can do a variety of interval workouts. If you're going to do interval training, you can program the heart rate monitor to chirp at a specific time period, say every five minutes. At each chirp you either increase your training intensity to your upper limit (145 bpm) or decrease your intensity to your lower limit (125 bpm). This type of interval workout allows you to crisscross the entire range of your TZ safely and efficiently.

Finally, the recovery phase of a workout is very important. I prefer to use a two minute recovery phase. When you have finished the workout, you press the stop watch button and the timer freezes that point. But the heart rate monitor continues to calculate a post-workout two minute period. The monitor will then post this time on one of the screens when you recall the data. You need to program the desired recovery period before you begin; a recovery period from 1–4 minutes is usually standard.

Once you have programmed your workout into the wrist monitor and strapped the monitor to your wrist, handlebars, treadmill bar, or wherever within a three foot radius you will be able to see the continuing read-out of your heart's activities, grab a partner and go. It works best if your partner's conditioning roughly matches your own. That way, you can stay together throughout the run.

Now, here's the tricky part. You need to monitor your monitor. That is, you must constantly make adjustments during your workout to make sure you're on target with your workout plan. This allows you to fine tune your training program. I like to set an alarm on my heart rate monitor to chirp every three or four minutes to remind me to take a look. After awhile this becomes a habit and takes very little effort.

But to continue with our example, after your six minute warm-up, you'll hear the chirp signalling you to begin your main set. Without even looking at your heart rate monitor, spend the next few minutes slowly accelerating your pace. Your partner says "36" aloud, which means they quickly looked at their display and their heart rate monitor reading is 136. You check yours and respond with a "31," dropping the "one hundred" for simplicity's sake. The chatter between the two of you might be something like this: "38," "35," "41," "41." Eventually one of you will hear the chirp signalling that you have reached the upper limits of your TZ, in this case 145.

When you reach this point, maintain this pace until you hear your heart rate monitor signal the programmed five minute interval. Reign back slightly and slowly reduce your intensity. As your heart rate drops, call it out: "41," "41" (pause for a minute), "34," "31." Continue until your heart rate monitor signals that you have reached the lower level of your TZ, 125 bpm.

Again you gradually accelerate and crisscross back and forth through your entire training zone (125-145 bpm). Exactly 48 minutes later you will hear the beep from the second alarm telling you that the main set is over and that it is time to cooldown. Relax and enjoy the cooldown until you hear the final chirp a few minutes later.

Advanced heart rate monitors can store all of the heart rate data during your workout. Later you can use the data to determine how long you trained in each of your five training zones.

AFTER YOUR WORKOUT:
COLLECTING HEART RATE MONITOR DATA

On high-end heart rate monitor models there are two ways of downloading workout information for your post-workout recall or retrieval.

Manually, you can push the recall button repeatedly and write down the heart rate and record it for each 5 or 15 or 60 seconds of the exercise period.That is, if you have the recording interval on 60 seconds and you worked out for 60 minutes you would have 60 different heart rate readings to write down. Then you can manually plot this data and graph it yourself on your own spreadsheet program or by hand. If you take the pencil and paper approach, this is how several minutes of data may look:

Time	Heart rate	Time	Heart rate
1	79	9	128
2	95	10	122
3	125	11	130
4	142	12	139
5	149	13	145
6	138	14	140
7	132	15	135
8	128	16	124

Now you may graph this information, roughly calculating your average heart rate, and noting your five minute training intervals. Or, you can download the data into a computer, as I discussed before and print a hard copy for your files.

For a sixty minute criss-cross heart rate monitor workout, a printout of the data should look something like this:

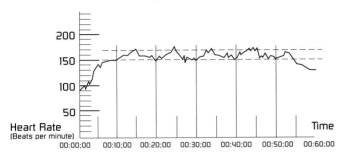

Racing with a wireless telemetry heart rate monitor can be worth milliseconds in a sprint, minutes in a marathon, and hours in an ultra. Training with a heart rate monitor can mean hundreds of calories burned, many pounds of fat lost, and shorter, more motivated and enjoyable workouts. Take the basics from this chapter and play with them, construct your own favorite workouts, and most of all, save this invaluable data to track your progress and refine your exercise program.

If you want to send me a letter and describe your favorite heart rate monitor workout, I'd love to hear from you, and I promise I'll write you back. I will even share the workout and credit you with it in the subsequent reprints of The Heart Rate Monitor Book. Write me c/o Fleet Feet, Inc., 2408 "J" Street, Sacramento, CA, 95816.

Soon you will find yourself performing at increasingly higher levels, as you come to understand the dynamic interaction between your mind and your body. Your body is the machine, your mind is the control room, and the heart rate monitor is the link between the two.

LADDERS, BEAT INTERVALS, GAME RACING, AND GEAR TESTING

Each winter Olympics, from 1976 through 1988, I represented the USA on our biathlon team, and simultaneously, I slowly transitioned from being an athlete to being a consultant and coach to cross-country skiers and fitness athletes. In 1984, when the first commercial wireless heart rate monitors were sold in the United States, I acquired one from what was probably one of the first shipments that were sent to retail stores. I have used them with almost religious commitment since that momentous day, when I became the excited owner of the most informative piece of equipment that an athlete can own.

I have dozens of favorite training sessions using my heart rate monitor, and each serves a specific purpose with my athletes' training programs. It was actually very hard to limit myself here to just these:

LADDERS

Ladders are ideal interval workouts for any sport; you can use them for skiing, running, cycling, aerobics, swimming, and so forth. This particular ladder we call the "five minutes, five beats per minute" ladder. Take your Max HR and subtract 40 bpm. Then after a warm-up, start at this low value, plus five beats for your initial zone, and go continuously for five minutes. If your heart rate monitor has a timer, set it for five minutes, and every time you hear the chirp from the alarm, "step up the ladder" and into the next five beat zone. Complete five steps up the ladder, and then descend the ladder by stepping down each five minutes into the next lower five beat zone. This is about a 45 minute (plus warm-up and cool-down) workout.

40 BEAT INTERVAL

This one is intense. Take your Max HR and subtract 50 bpm from that number. Warm up until you are comfortable, then begin by continuously (but slowly) picking up the pace until your monitor indicates that you are at your Max HR less 10 beats. Then, back off the pace until you are back down, 40 bpm lower, at your Max HR minus 50 beats. If you have a heart rate monitor which can be programmed with an alarm sound, set these values into the alarm and perform the whole workout by having your heart rate monitor signal when to pick it up and when to drop down again by 40 beats. Example: Your Max HR is 180 bpm. Subtract 50 beats and start the interval at 130, slowly increasing the intensity until you reach 170 bpm, then back off and continue to ease off on the intensity until you see 130 again. Billy Koch, America's all-time best cross-country skier, uses a 90 beat interval for this workout.

GAME RACING

Because I coach on the weekends and travel with my athletes, I don't have the chance to enter races anymore. I still love to race though, so I have designated Wednesdays to be my race days, and I have set three different race courses of three different lengths to use. Since I don't have fellow athletes to compete against, I have traded them for my heart rate monitor, which now becomes not only my motivator, but also my competitor.

My goal is to run at an even heart rate pace throughout the distance. Because of the training effect, if my training program is working, my heart rate response should gradually come down. Let's take my Wednesday 25k bike time trial. I plug into an even heart rate pace of 160 bpm and when I get to the finishline my finish time is 65 minutes. Two weeks later I repeat the race, and my finish time at the same heart rate level is 64 minutes. From all this I gain two things: an excellent workout at 85% of my Max HR, and the knowledge that my training program is on target. I am getting fitter, faster, and more efficient.

GEAR TESTING

Over the years, I have helped a number of equipment manufacturers with the design and development of their gear. They are usually inventor-engineer types who like to put their products through tests on machines for strength, adhesion, and wear and tear. They ask me to test the gear for true field response, for performance, and I tell them that the most valid performance test for efficiency and speed is an athlete.

For example, if I were testing a new pair of Specialized Composite wheels, I'd test them against what I have been using to see if they perform as well or better. The way I'd do it would be to give the equipment a heart rate monitor test. I would take a ride with one set of wheels at a fixed heart rate, usually 80% of Max HR. Then, two or so days later, on the same course and under the same personal (sleep, nutrition) and environmental conditions, I'd do the same with the second set. I usually repeat these tests about five times and average the results to find out which piece of equipment is faster. You can perform this test for more than just gear. It works as a great test for your biomechanics. Test different positions of your arms on a bike, or change your running form and take the test. You'll learn a lot about your gear and your form by training using a heart rate monitor as the true laboratory testing equipment.

Using a heart rate monitor, you can test different pieces of training equipment. Here Matthew Brick tests different handlebars to determine the ones that work best for him.

Lyle Nelson is a partner in Rudolph and Nelson, an events marketing and consulting company headquartered in Portland, Oregon. They produce the Kingsbery Summer Biathlon Series as well as numerous other events. Lyle is a personal coach to several world-class biathletes, writes numerous articles, and is a motivational speaker. The highlight of his career was carrying the USA flag into the opening Olympic ceremonies during the 1988 Olympics in Calgary. He can be reached at PO Box 997, Portland, Oregon 97207 or (503) 721-0181.

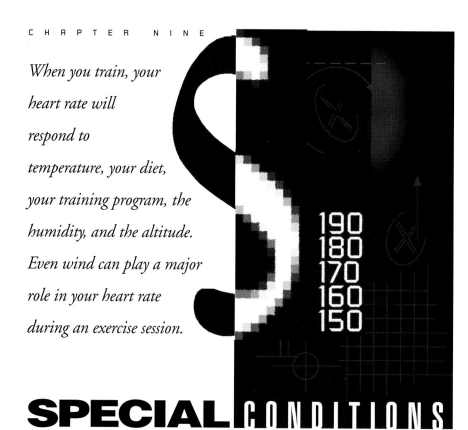

CHAPTER NINE

When you train, your heart rate will respond to temperature, your diet, your training program, the humidity, and the altitude. Even wind can play a major role in your heart rate during an exercise session.

190
180
170
160
150

SPECIAL CONDITIONS

Your heart rate monitor reflects your body's reaction to all variables. If you are anxious or suffering from a lack of sleep, your heart rate will be elevated. Likewise, if you are training in 100 degree heat, your entire body will be adjusting to that. With the number of factors involved, an athlete's performance on any given day can often seem as predictable as the lottery.

Luckily, the heart rate monitor doesn't have to check the temperature or psychoanalyze anybody. All it has to do is give you the bottom line, consistently and accurately. And the bottom line is your heart rate, your body's reaction to everything within and without.

Here are a number of factors, environmental and otherwise, that impact the performance of every athlete—whether professional or amateur.

ALTITUDES: HIGH AND LOW

There has been a lot of research done with athletes training and racing at varying altitudes, and the bottom line is that your response to altitude is directly related to how long you've been at that particular altitude, with most athletes adjusting at about the same rate.

If you live at sea level and you train above 6,000 feet (or about 1,800 m) for the first time, your heart rate will slow somewhat. After several hours,

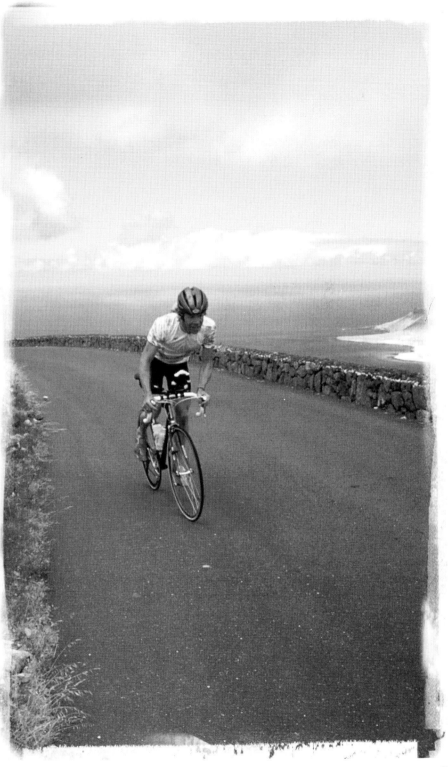

however, this trend reverses itself and your heart rate rises about 10% above your Resting HR. If you continue your journey upward, say to heights over 10,000 feet (about 3,000 m), your Resting HR can increase to 50% higher than normal.

This increased heart rate lasts for several days while your system adjusts to the lower oxygen concentrations in the air outside (causing you to breathe more breaths per minute) and to the lower air pressure (the air pressure inside your lungs is therefore also lower, which causes the amount of oxygen in your lungs to be lower, too). Then, slowly, your Resting HR drops back down to your sea level heart rate. All in all, the process takes about 14 days. This adaptation process is called acclimatization, and graphed out, it looks like this:

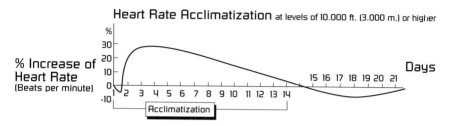

Training at newly introduced, higher altitudes can be very deceiving. You may think you are running an 8 minute mile, while in actuality you're running at an 8 1/2 minute pace. Were you to train according to pace and not heart rate, you would be beyond your heart rate training zone without even knowing it.

You can actually keep track of your acclimatization changes yourself. The next time you stay for an extended time at a new altitude, write down your Resting HR every morning. It's kind of fun to watch that number drop each day. Your body is making adjustments, respiratory, metabolic, and physiological changes, to make up for the conditions at higher altitudes. To compensate for thinner air and for the lower atmospheric pressure, your body makes more red blood cells and more hemoglobin so you can transport more oxygen. This increase in red blood cells in turn increases several other important things: the amount of blood that your heart pumps out (your cardiac output), the circulation in the local blood vessels, and other cellular functions such as the numbers of mitochondria and aerobic enzymes.

If you are a flatlander and you travel to the mountains with a friend who lives at a moderate altitude, your friend has a definite training advantage over you. They are already partially acclimatized and you aren't. Don't let this get you down, but also don't think that you can go up to a higher altitude, train, and then return to lower altitudes and race better. It doesn't quite work that easily.

It seems like training at a high altitude which increases an athlete's hemoglobin and gives the athlete higher concentrations of certain enzymes, would therefore increasing her/his performance at lower altitudes. Unfortunately, the body adapts very quickly to drops in altitude so training of this sort actually has very little impact on one's athletic performance.

If you are an endurance athlete, here's one more note. Above 5,000 feet (1,500 m), your max VO2 drops regardless of acclimatization. The rate of this drop is 2% for every 1,000 feet (300 m) of altitude.

TEMPERATURE CHANGES: HOT AND COLD

This marvelous organism we call a body has an amazing ability to automatically adapt to its surroundings. Temperature adaptations are an ideal example of this, because the changes are so readily apparent.

When you exercise, muscle activity produces heat which raises your body temperature. Your body's primary goal, in response to temperature changes, is to maintain equilibrium of your core or deeper tissue's temperatures. This is called thermal balance. When hot, your body dissipates heat through physiological changes—a process called heat regulation. An increased heart rate, increased blood flow to the skin, and sweating (as much as 1–1.5 gallons [3.6–5.4 liters] per hour) are all part of the heat regulation process.

In cold conditions, your body tries to increase your core temperature by lowering the amount of blood flow to anything but your core. The body also shivers, which causes a three- to five-fold increase in your metabolic rate and heat production. Finally, hormones are released which cause an overall increase in your basal metabolic rate as well.

There is a direct relationship between temperature changes and heart rates: the higher the temperature, the higher the heart rate. I performed a test on this correlation myself. Using my heart rate monitor, I ventured into a sauna (set at 120 fahrenheit) to watch my heart rate respond to the sudden temperature change. Here's what happened:

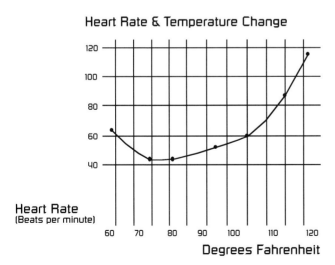

Heart Rate & Temperature Change

Heart Rate
(Beats per minute)

Degrees Fahrenheit

This isn't really Nobel Prize research material, but it's fun to test a theory on yourself. What this graph tells us is what we all pretty much know, the higher the ambient temperature, the higher the resting heart rate.

When you train in hot weather, your body's normal responses to heat are compounded by your heat-producing muscle activity, so your heart works harder still to cool your body, and the end result is an elevated heart rate. Again, use your heart rate, not your stop watch, when working out in heat. You need to pay attention if your heart rate monitor is telling you to take it easy.

The ideal temperature for training depends on the type of exercise. If you are performing sprint-like activities, those of short duration and high power requirements, the ideal dry air temperature is between 75-95 degrees F (25-35 C). For easier, longer activities the ideal ambient temperature is 68 degrees F (20 degrees C).

Heat adaptation comes from exercising regularly in hot conditions. These adjustments, or acclimatizations, usually take about 10 days of heat training. Among the adaptations are improved blood flow from the deep tissues to the skin, heart rate increases, lower temperature sweat break-point, increased perspiration, and a decreased sweat salt content.

Heat adaptation and tolerance to heat do not change much with age. Nor does heat adaptation vary significantly based on gender.

The body does not go through such dramatic changes during cold acclimatization. For athletes of any sort, it is much easier to adjust to moderately cold temperatures by simply wearing the right kind of clothing. Still, when considering cold temperatures, don't forget about the wind chill factor; 30 degrees at 25 mph is a lot different than 30 degrees at a slow trot.

DEHYDRATION

Remember those old movies with tattered Legionnaires crawling across the desert, mouths full of sand, footprints disappearing into the horizon? "Water..." they croaked, "..water." I've felt like that before. Of course, all I had to do was reach down for a water bottle or stop at a drinking faucet, but those miserable soldiers always come to mind when I start dehydrating. I know it's a bit strange, but what's life without a little drama?

You don't have to be in a desert to dehydrate. In fact, you can dehydrate in cold conditions as well (the harder you breathe, the more water escapes through the respiratory passages). Sweating obviously depletes your body of water and salts, so if your body starts running low on liquids, your heart is forced to work harder. Here's what happens to your heart rate if you don't drink enough replacement fluids:

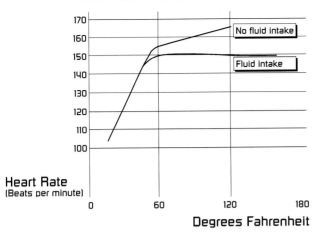

Heart Rate & Temperature Change

No fluid intake

Fluid intake

Heart Rate
(Beats per minute)

Degrees Fahrenheit

As you become increasingly dehydrated, your total blood volume drops. Because the heart has access to less blood, it must pump faster to circulate the same amount of blood, diverting needed performance energy from your other muscles.

The message is clear. You need to drink frequently to maintain your blood volume when you train. There are so many factors that determine how much and how often you should drink that absolute rules on the subject are unwise to offer. Roughly though, you need to increase your intake of fluids to five or six times normal when you exercise. For marathon runners, fluid losses can reach levels of 1.5 gallons (5.4 liters) per hour. The same is true of football players, wrestlers, skiers, and other high intensity athletes. If you don't replace these fluids, your heart rate will increase, and your ability to perform will decrease rapidly.

FOOD

I must admit, some food I've had the displeasure of consuming actually raised my heart rate before I took a bite. Call it "anticipatory nausea" if you will. This section, however, deals with what happens after the food enters your system.

Consider food to be your body's fuel source. Unfortunately, there are no labels reading "Unleaded Only" or "Diesel Only" stamped across your lips, letting you know what kind of food your body prefers. Still, by using your heart rate monitor, it is pretty easy to determine what kinds of foods you should be eating before, during, and after your training.

In 1986, a group of world-class triathletes were invited to participate in the longest endurance study ever performed. Doug Hiller, M.D. and Mary O'Toole, Ph.D. used their laboratory at the University of Tennessee (at a cost of about $20,000 per athlete) to answer some specific endurance questions.

They stuck us with an 8 hour workout which included simulated swimming with a hand crank, cycling on a bicycle ergometer, and running on a treadmill.

All activities were done at 75% of each of our Max HR. They stuck gas analyzers in our mouths and heparin locks in both of our arms, scraped us frequently for sweat samples, measured our core body temperatures, collected our urine, controlled our calorie input, and controlled the air temperature. Nearly every function of our body was under a microscope for 8 hours.

What they learned was fascinating and very applicable to my training program. First, the results showed that all of us burned both carbohydrates and fats as fuel sources throughout the experiment, but each of our bodies automatically selected its own ratio of fat calories and carbohydrate calories used. I, for example, am an 80% carbo burner and a 20% fat burner. On the other hand, there were others in the test who were much closer to being 80% fat burners and 20% carbo burners. I now know which fuel sources to ingest when I race and train—carbohydrates.

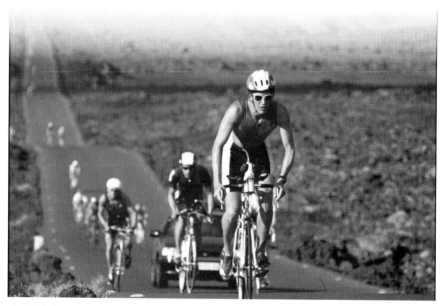

At high intensity levels, heart rate monitors are an essential piece of racing equipment

Secondly, I learned that I was extremely low in sodium and that I needed to sodium-load before a hard race. I also needed to increase the amount of sodium in my diet. I had bought into the popular anti-salt fad that took table salt off America's dining tables and out of our kitchens. Bunk. If you are an endurance athlete, you need salt in your diet. Because I am a vegetarian, I need even more because there isn't a lot of salt in the foods I eat.

Your heart rate monitor can help you determine which kinds of food your body best metabolizes. In a sense, you're using your heart rate monitor as a miniature exercise testing laboratory.

THE BEST FUEL TEST

Eat a high carbohydrate meal. Wait 1-2 hours, then time yourself on your completion of a controlled workout of a distance (like a 20-25 mile [40-45k] bike ride or a 6-9 mile [10-15k] run) that takes about an hour or so at 75-80% Max HR, with no wind and ambient temperatures of 60-75 degrees. Record your heart rate before, during, and after the workout at pre-set intervals. Also remember how much and what kind of fluids you drink during the workout, so that you can repeat your same fluid use when you complete the workout again for comparison. When you are done, write down your elapsed time and rest for several days.

Then, several days later, eat a high fat meal. Wait 1-2 hours and complete the same workout, keeping all variables such as distance, temperature, and fluid usage the same as previously. Carefully log the elapsed time. Now, graph your heart rates over the entire workout. Notice which food produced the faster times and lower heart rates. It should be readily apparent which fuel source works best for you.

The longer the workout, the more your nutritional choices begin to affect your performance. You can discover your optimal workout diet by using your heart rate monitor to perform tests similar to the one outlined above with different food choices.

You can also perform a "during training fuel source" test. Drink only 100% glucose drinks during a race and measure your heart rates. On another day, drink a mixture of glucose and fat combined and see what your heart rate response is. Don't forget to try different companies' products during simulated racing conditions and test them based on heart rate.

In laboratory tests, the amount of improvement between one fuel source and another can be as high as 7%. That is a considerable difference—certainly enough to justify further explorations into your personal nutritional needs.

ILLNESS/OVERTRAINING

For many athletes, heart rate monitors can be used as an alarm that alerts them that they are training at intensities, frequencies, or durations beyond levels which improve performance. Overtraining is a common mistake, especially among athletes who believe more is better and don't take a systematic approach to training.

One of the best indications of over-training is your morning Resting HR. If this before-you-get-out-of-bed heart rate is 10 beats per minute higher than normal, you need to be concerned. An accelerated Resting HR could indicate any number of problems: you may be overtraining, suffering from fatigue, slightly injured, or even fighting off a fever or a stress-related problem.

Rest is one of the best medicines that an athlete can use. Unfortunately, it's one of the toughest to prescribe, because many athletes fear deconditioning. The facts are that deconditioning, the loss of fitness, does not occur until you remain inactive for a minimum of four days. So what do a couple of days off really matter? No one is getting ahead of you, unless you let them by running yourself into serious downtime due to illness, injury, or psychological frustrations.

You must always keep a balance and listen to your body. If it wants to rest, then take a couple of days off. If it performs better with carbohydrates, then have a spaghetti feast. The key is to use your mind to improve your training habits and enhance your body's performance. Once you use the heart rate monitor as the link between your mind and your body, they will start to respect each other's needs and states. From this stems an understanding of the true nature of performance.

USING HEART RATE MONITORS UNDER SPECIAL CONDITIONS

From our experience at Georgia State University, Atlanta, we have found heart rate monitors useful in a variety of situations. Here are four examples:

1. Athletes who "yo-yo" to and from high altitudes and sea level.

Kenny Souza, for example, lives in Boulder, but he may find it necessary to stay in his native California for a week or two for racing or other reasons. If he is doing a track session, say 4 x 1,500m or 6 x 1,000m, as a long interval day, the pace he needs to run for optimum development will be slower at 6,000 feet in Boulder than it will at sea level in California. We use heart rate as an indicator of effort, and Kenny would vary his pace appropriately. Our periodic treadmill test data tell us the heart rate he needs for optimum training effect, and he need only glance at his heart rate monitor to check on his running intensity. Pace then becomes secondary.

2. Monitoring the cardiac stress of very long training runs done in warm weather when fluid losses from sweating are sizable.

We know that cardiac output is the product of heart rate and stroke volume. For example, during a 25 mile run in 80 degree weather, even though fluids are ingested, the athlete will be in negative fluid balance. This will tend to decrease plasma volume. As this continues, the only way that cardiac output can be maintained is for heart rate to rise, since stroke volume is decreasing due to the reduced blood volume. Often, athletes get almost entranced into a given cadence and pace, and even though they sense greater effort, they tend to hold pace. This may be acceptable in a race, provided they do not become a medical casualty. But if the object of the run is

FROM EXPERIENCE
DAVID MARTIN, PhD.
FROM EXPERIENCE

an easy but long training effort, we need to slow the pace in the later stages to keep the equivalent stress fairly constant. Heart rate monitoring permits this.

3. Long training runs with long uphill segments.

Runners often tend instinctively to maintain a level pace when climbing hills, working harder in the process and often going anaerobic during their aerobic day. Wearing a heart rate monitor can eliminate this. If the session is to be done at between 140 and 145 bpm, as the uphill climb raises the heart rate to 155, the heart rate monitor can alert the runner to this and she or he can then slow their pace, keeping the hill climb as conversational and pleasant as the level section just completed.

4. Assessing changes in fitness over time.

A session of 6 x 1 mile track repeats done in early March may give an athlete results of 4:35 per mile, with a heart rate of 185 bpm. A month later, with similar weather conditions, the 6 x 1 mile session now sees 4:35 mile repeats done with a heart rate of only 175 bpm, or mile repeats of 4:25 being managed with a heart rate of 185. This suggests an improvement of fitness and can give a factual accompaniment to athletes' comments along the lines of "You know, with this April mile repeat session it seemed easier to run at the same pace as it did a month ago; in fact, I could probably have run faster, and I wouldn't have been any more tired than a month ago at a slower pace."

David Martin is Regents Professor of Health Sciences in the Department of Cardiopulmonary Care Sciences at Georgia State University. He has worked with elite athletes for over twenty-five years, is the author of Training Distance Runners (1991), chairperson of TAC's Sport Sciences, and coaches and advises elite-level runners and duathletes.

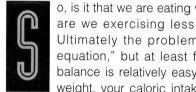

Heart Rate Monitor Diet Plan

The United States might have stopped adding territory a long time ago, but it certainly hasn't stopped expanding. Americans, on average, gain one pound a year after age 20. In fifteen years you can gain fifteen pounds of body weight, and most of that is fat. I'll let you work out your own numbers if you want (it can be a little depressing for anyone over 35).

So, is it that we are eating worse and/or more and gaining weight? Or, are we exercising less, eating the same and gaining weight? Ultimately the problem can be on either side of the "fitness equation," but at least figuring out where the equation is out of balance is relatively easy. Simply, in order to maintain your current weight, your caloric intake must equal your caloric usage. You will eventually gain or lose weight depending upon which side of the equation you're partial towards. It has long been shown that working with the fitness equation is the only real, reliable way to attain long-term weight loss.

Looking at recent dietary studies, the overall American dietary trend shows a definite shift from quantity to quality. That is, as a nation, we are eating better (but not perfectly, or all the fast food and dessert manufacturers would be out of business) and less. Unfortunately, we are also burning fewer calories than we have historically. The bottom line: we are eating better, exercising less, and gaining weight along the way.

A heart rate monitor can be one of the most important tools that you can use if you want to lose weight. By properly setting your training level, you can maximize your ability to burn off the right kind of calories. Different foods (fuels) burn off at different intensity levels, in much the same way as vehicles

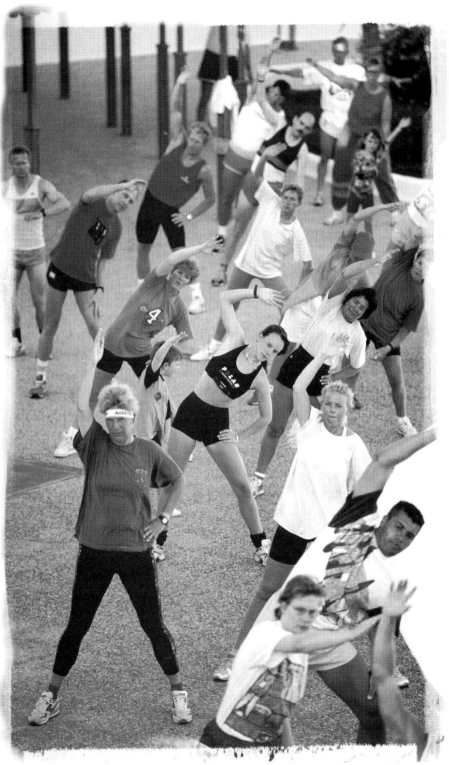

burn their fuels. For example, high performance cars require extremely high octane fuels to achieve speeds above 120 mph, and the body needs high octane carbohydrates (complex sugars) to achieve the same sort of maximal performance. Meanwhile, 18 wheel trucks are carrying big loads, moving down the road slowly, and are tanked up with diesel fuel. Fat is the diesel fuel of the human body.

You've probably heard somewhere by now that while one gram of fat contains nine calories, one gram of carbohydrate contains only four calories. This is important to remember, because in terms of the weight of the food you eat, one gram of fat is the same as one gram of carbohydrate, and yet it delivers over 100% more calories.

The following is key: fat burns slowly, but it burns in higher amounts if the exercise intensity is low. Carbohydrates burn at a faster rate and are the body's first fuel source if there is a high intensity demand. Both types of fuel, fats and carbs, are always burning simultaneously, it is the proportion of the two that varies.

As an example, if you are of average fitness and body weight, when you are walking at a 15 minute per mile (9 minute per kilometer) pace, you are burning more than 50% of your calories from fat sources (fat molecules that come from either recent dietary sources or from your own stored body fat). When you pick up the pace, your body starts to burn a higher concentration of carbohydrates (broken down into glycogen). The winning formula, if you are exercising to lose weight, is simple: go slow and go long.

Covert Bailey, in his now classic book Fit or Fat, first introduced the concept of carbohydrates as the twigs in a fire that burn very quickly and at high intensities. He then showed that fat burns at low intensities, much like a big log in a fire. It takes the twigs to get the log burning, but once you have it started, the log burns long and warm and needs few if any additional twigs to continue going. Again, visualize the carbohydrate twigs as being consumed in the hot fire of high intensity (high bpm) exercise, then imagine those fat logs burning in long, low intensity, low bpm workouts.

The heart rate monitor will help keep you in the mode of burning a higher proportion of fat calories if you set your training levels properly. The most important factors to remember when training to lose weight are to go slowly, go continuously, go moderately, and most importantly, GO!

There is one important fact for you to remember. The higher heart rate the more total calories you will burn. That is if you train slowly, you will burn more fat calories but less total calories than if you train harder, at a higher heart rate.

There has been some misunderstanding between burning more fat and burning more calories as was just explained. Exercising at a lower heart rate or a lower intensity requires less "quick" energy or calories from carbohydrates. By training on the lower end of the scale such as the Weight Management Zone which is 60-70% of your Max HR an even higher number of calories from fat sources burned. But, there are fewer total calories being utilized at the same time.

Even though at the lower heart rates you are burning a higher percentage of fat, a lower total amount of fat is lost because there is a lower amount of total calories burned. This is to say that over the same amount of exercise time, you will burn more calories at higher heart rate zones. The key to this seeming dilemma is quite simple: the length of time that you exercise. The easier that you go in terms of heart rates, the longer time you need to commit to and the reciprocal is just as true. When you train in the lower heart rate zones you still burn a significant number of calories but only over a period of time.

There is no doubt among the experts that optimum weight loss is achieved through exercise in the Weight Management Zone. But, the length of exercise time must be long and it needs to be regular and frequent. Here´s a good exemple: a golfer (without a cart) plays three hours of golf and burns about 900 calories. An average sized runner puts in 30 minutes of running and burns about 400 calories. If they each play three times a week the golfer burns more total calories and thus the golfer would lose more weight than the runner who runs three times a week.

Over the years, the rule of thumb for exercise to achieve maximum benefit has been to train at 65-70% of your Max HR. But, that advice has changed drastically in the last few years. The American College of Sports Medicine (ACSM) has dropped there recommendations concerning exercise intensity because they know that very low-intensity or heart rates can be extremely beneficial, especially in longterm weight loss programs. Rather, they now say that the length of time you exercise not the intensity level is the key factor to our health. It appears that 35 minutes (not 20 minutes) seems to produce the greatest improvements.

When you set out to exercise to lose fat, you now know that not only do you have to exercise at a lower heart rate to lose weight, you also have to work out with physical activities that are easy to do and continuous in nature, so examine your choices of activities carefully. Take tennis. You would think that by playing a good game of tennis that you could lose some weight.

First, you hit the ball and rally it several times before the point is won or lost. The average length of time of a rally is about ten seconds, which represents about four hits total. The length of time from serve to serve is about

60 seconds. That means that tennis is an interval activity which requires high heart rates during the playing time and continuous, low heart rate rest during the between play periods.

During a recent men's four set Wimbledon match, the game lasted over four hours, and yet the ball was only in the air for nine minutes. During those nine minutes of all-out effort, the players' heart rates soared, only to plunge downward during the rest interval. This obviously goes against our go slow, go long maxim. Thus, tennis is a dud for weight loss activities.

Look for sports that require continuous activity, those that require lower heart rates, and those that last over a long period of time. Simply, you want exercise activities that are easy, fun, and that take up a chunk of time. Here's a list of some of them: walking (fast or slow depending upon your conditioning and target heart rate), aerobics, jogging/running, cycling (stationary bikes), snowshoeing, rowing, dancing, racquetball, handball, squash, in-line skating, and cross-country skiing. Even hitting a punching bag works if done correctly, as a low intensity workout.

Sorry, but golf, sex, and tennis are duds. They are all interval activities, and in the case of sex, the amount of time spent in the aerobic fitness threshold zone (usually about 10-15 seconds for men at 110-130 bpm) is disappointingly brief. Golf and tennis don't fit the category of moderate exercise either. Golf is fun, but it's a sports game, not a fitness sport.

One last word about sex. Forget the rally call of "reach for your mate instead of the plate." That was the myth that drove a weight loss movement a few years ago. It was fun, but ineffective. The idea was that if you turned to sex instead of food, you would curb your appetite. Sex doesn't curb your appetite, if anything, it makes you hungrier. Granted, its difficult to eat while engaged in such activity, but it is by definition an interval sport.

HERE'S THE BOTTOM LINE ON WEIGHT LOSS:

1. Eat fewer calories than you will burn.

2. Eat complex carbohydrates (i.e., bananas, rice, potatoes, pasta, and apples), because for the same weight of food you are eating less than half the calories.

3. Eliminate "empty calories" (i.e., refined sugars such as those in candy bars and soft drinks, corn syrup, and cornstarch) from your meals, as they contribute nothing to your diet.

4. Exercise slow and long, for at least 30 minutes a day, five days a week, at your Moderate Activity or Weight Management training zone intensities (50-70% Max HR). This will burn more of your body's fat calories than your stored carbohydrate calories.

It's that simple. So put that $20 you were going to spend on your next diet book towards a long term, life enhancing investment like a heart rate monitor. I can't guarantee that you'll lose 40 pounds in a month, but I can say that you'll feel much better about yourself if you lose weight while increasing your personal fitness level. Believe me, exercise and a healthy lifestyle can be even more addicting than chocolate and twice as sweet in the long run.

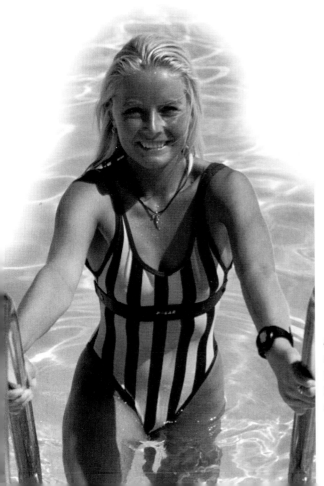

Swimming is a good way of staying lean. The workout intensity is easy to monitor with a heart rate monitor.

"EXERCISE SAVED MY LIFE"

Shortly after midnight on July 23, 1990, Lauren Bergen, then 38, rushed herself to the emergency room of a New York City hospital. Her heart was racing, and she was gasping for breath. One look at her 280 pound, 5' 2" frame, told the attending physician that if she wasn't having a heart attack right then and there, she was at prime risk for one in the near future.

It turned out that the evening's episode was not a heart attack, but an extreme allergic reaction to caffeine. It didn't make a difference to Lauren, though. She was frightened enough by the experience to decide that it was time to take action, and she began a total lifestyle change.

Lauren joined a weight loss support group and a fitness center and was told by her trainers that she needed to keep track of her pulse, before, during, and after her workouts. Unfortunately, the layers of fat on her wrists made it almost impossible for her to take her pulse manually, and if she was able to find it, it took so long that her heart rate had dropped dramatically.

Just about then, Lauren read an article about the use of heart rate monitors in weight loss programs, and she immediately called the company to arrange overnight delivery of one for her. She then was able to establish target heart rate zones for her workouts and keep track of her progress in a training diary. Soon Lauren was going for time and endurance in her exercise, and her resting heart rate dropped steadily to the mid-50s, from a high of 93. Lauren's excess weight has come off steadily, at a rate of two to three pounds each week, and her dress size has gone from a 30 to a 12.

Lauren works out six days a week for about two hours per day, keeping her exercising heart rate in the 130-140 range (about 60% of her Max HR), which she says has worked perfectly to shed her excess pounds. Because she now finds exercise to be fun again, she also swims (her heart rate monitor is water resistant) and takes aerobics classes, where she says, "The Polar monitor is excellent, because the training level in 'step,' as well as traditional aerobics classes must be monitored carefully."

The advice Lauren gives to others who are seriously overweight is to apply mind over matter and to go about the rehabilitation process purposefully. "It must become a way of life," she declares, "and to do it sensibly you need a lot of help and the right technology."

Lauren notes that the process of losing weight also has very nice surprise dividends. Recently, she was pulled over by a police officer for exceeding the speed limit. When she produced her driver's license, the officer looked and looked at the picture, not believing that the photo could be of the woman in front of him. Finally, after a last hard look, the officer returned the license, saying only, "Keep up the good work."

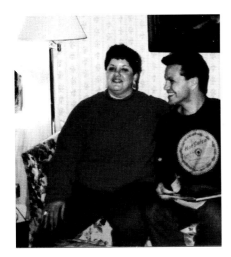

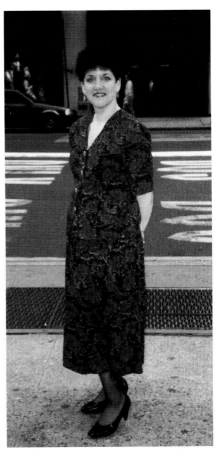

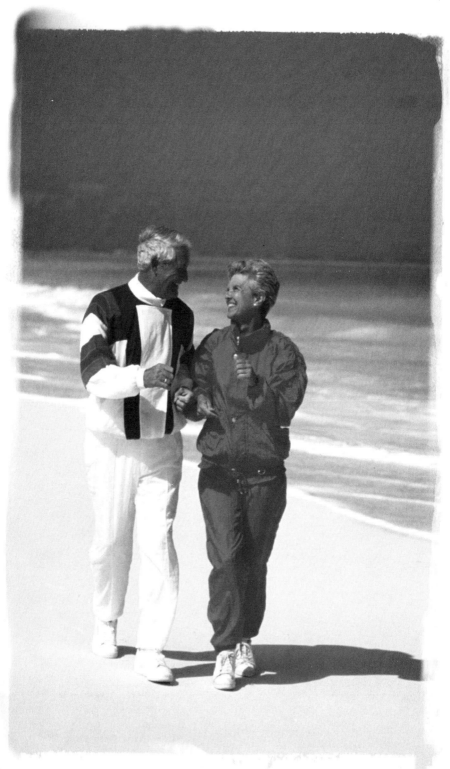

Cardiac REHABILITATION

Most people don't think of their hearts very often; it's there, and it's obviously working. But if their hearts didn't work, even for a moment, there would be little question that something was drastically wrong. Your heart beats more than 100,000 times a day, 3 million times a month or 36 million times a year, and your survival depends on its consistency and performance.

nd yet, this powerful muscle pump and its arteries sometimes fail us. Coronary artery disease and myocardial infarctions kill more people in the United States than any other diseases or ailments. And even though it has been shown that cardiac rehabilitation programs work, only about 100,000 US citizens per year (of the estimated 5.7 million who suffer from some form of heart disease) are participating in these programs.

Cardiac physicians have long been prescribing exercise as a part of cardiac rehabilitation, and since the early 1960's, when cardiac rehabilitation became more prevalent, cardiac rehab patients who exercise have been doing consistently better than those who do not. But, rehabilitation patients' programs must be carefully planned and monitored for a safe recovery. That's where heart rate monitors come in.

THE CARDIAC REHABILITATION PROGRAM

Cardiac rehab patients can benefit from walking, lifting (with supervision), or even just sitting up in bed. No matter what phase a cardiac patient is in, she or he can do something to improve their muscle tone, heart, and lung function, and generally improve their mood and decrease their anxiety. Even walking to the mailbox each day can resemble a rehabilitation program for a coronary heart disease patient.

There are some patients who should not participate in comprehensive cardiac rehabilitation programs. There is a great deal of controversy surrounding this process of determination. However, all cardiac patients should be eligible for selected cardiac rehabilitation services (e.g. patient education, exercise therapy, risk-factor modification) to potentially prevent a deterioration in risk status over time.

For those participating in a rehab program, the safety issue is foremost. It can be reassuring to remember, however, that fewer than one cardiac event occurs for every 80,000 hours of exercise.

A medically supervised outpatient rehabilitation program is the best treatment for cardiac patients. However, many patients do not have or take the opportunity to participate in supervised rehabilitation programs due to lack of program availability, financial and health insurance situations, and other concerns. Home activity programs are feasible and beneficial for many low-risk cardiac patients. Even higher risk coronary patients may exercise at home after careful screening. Self-monitoring with a heart rate monitor is essential for these individuals. Of course, in addition they need periodic rehabilitation clinic visits, periodic primary physician visits, and transtelephonic ECG transmissions.

When designing a rehabilitation program, consideration must be given to the patient's individual needs: health history, medical status, severity of the disease, functional capacity, and stage of convalescence. Goals need to be established that are achievable and realistic considering the patient's limitations imposed by the disease.

Cardiac rehabilitation programs generally consist of four phases. They are as follows:

PHASE I = The hospitalized inpatient period. During this period, ordinarily 6–14 days, rehabilitation takes the form of both education (with discussion and counseling) and physical therapy. Therapy should be limited to range-of-motion activities: sitting, standing, walking. The main purpose is to reduce deconditioning caused by the long period of bed rest.

PHASE II = The convalescent period. During this 12 week period after hospital discharge, the exercise therapy begins. Ideally, the period begins within three weeks of hospital discharge. Patients are classified in one of three risk categories based on medical history, graded exercise test results, and other information relative to low, moderate, or high-risk patients. There is continuation of the education and lifestyle behavioral training.

PHASE III = The extended, supervised, outpatient program. This is a 4–6 month period which takes place after stabilized cardiovascular and physiological responses to exercise have been obtained.

PHASE IV = The ongoing lifetime unsupervised maintenance period. During this period, the patients use exercise therapy for lifestyle support—almost as a social outlet. Activities such as volleyball, walking or running, and dancing keep the patient's interest high and their exercise consistent. The emphasis can be more on activity rather than exercise.

Patients may move back and forth through these four phases as the disease regresses, progresses, or remains unchanged. But, the goal of a cardiac rehab program is independence and to see patients learn the self-monitoring skills that lead to independence. It is the rehab specialist's job to see the heart patient make the transition from direct medical supervision to reduced medical surveillance, through providing maximum safety, education, exercise guidelines, and sign and symptom monitoring.

The most effective forms of exercise for a cardiac patient are those that meet the following criteria:

- are aerobic
- use large muscle groups
- are maintained continuously
- are within an easy target heart rate zone
- build skeletal muscle strength

Forms of exercise which meet these five criteria include: jogging, walking, running, stationary or outdoor bicycling, swimming, skipping rope, rowing, climbing stairs, stepping on and off a bench, calisthenics, arm exercise, and weight training. Guidelines for the specifics of these programs are in part determined by the risk stratification, whether low, moderate, or high. Patients with coronary artery disease should avoid extremely vigorous exercise.

Training intensity is probably the single most important factor for a cardiac rehabilitation patient. Heart rate monitors can give such patients continuous, reliable feedback to aid in their recovery. Target heart rate intensities ranging from as low as 40%, but more typically between 60–80%, of symptom-limited Max HR are usually prescribed. It is best to choose the lower intensities and increase the duration of the workouts to achieve the desired training effect.

Specific formulas for heart rate intensities based on symptom-limited Max HR formulas have been calculated and are available from cardiac rehab specialists. Symptom-limited Max HR is that heart rate before abnormal signs and symptoms begin to occur.

Exercise intensity should never be higher than the patient's threshold for angina or ST segmental ischemic changes and never at a high level in the presence of known complex arrhythmias. Heart rate monitors are crucial in allowing patients to easily monitor their heart rates and can be used to alert patients if their heart rates go above prescribed levels. Heart rate monitors are also critical to coronary artery disease patients because for many the pressure from counting their pulse by pressing on their carotid artery (carotid palpating) can be dangerous and lead to the serious problem of carotid sinus reflex action.

Medications prescribed for management of cardiovascular conditions affect exercise testing and training. It's usually recommended that exercise testing for diagnostic purposes be carried out with the patient taking their prescribed drug treatments. Among the different cardiac medications, beta blockers have the greatest effect on exercise prescriptions. Beta blockers may not directly interfere with the positive effects of exercise therapy, but they can limit peak heart rate to 50% to 60% of the predicted maximum HR, and this may be an obstacle in achieving some of the benefits of higher intensity exercise.

CARDIAC REHABILITATION AND HEART RATE MONITORING: PHASE II PROGRAMS

The first step, in Phase II, is to define the patient's level of risk: low, moderate or high. This risk stratification is based on the patient's medical history, test results and other information.

Next, the patient needs a written exercise therapy prescription. The exercise prescription should come from the patient's cardiac rehab nurse or the exercise physiologist. The exercise prescription may be formulated after the patient performs an entrance graded exercise test and after risk stratification. For some patients, the risk of a graded exercise test is greater than the information gained, so they will not take the test.

The exercise prescription should include a minimum of three training sessions per week to obtain any real benefits, with four or even five exercise sessions per week perhaps being optimum. The length of time for the exercise therapy should be 15-60 minutes. This Phase II program always includes emergency support, direct professional supervision, and ECG monitoring. Each patient's exercise prescription should be reviewed and updated with regard to intensity, activity, and duration each week.

Generally, in Phase II, patients in formal cardiac rehabilitation programs are monitored with continuous electrocardiographic (ECG) telemetry monitoring. Most experts feel that ECG monitoring is essential to the safety and effectiveness of a prescribed regiment of exercise although it is an expensive procedure.

During the last two weeks of Phase II supervised programs, both ECG radiotelemetry systems and heart rate monitors may be used. The purpose of this dual protocol is to train patients on how to use and how to trust a heart rate monitor. Patients should be taught the full range of components of heart rate monitoring, including the various target heart rate zones, recovery heart rates, and resting heart rates. Then, when the patient advances to the Phase III maintenance exercise program, they can use their heart rate monitor to replace their ECG radiotelemetry system.

As the patient responds to the adaptation of exercise training, serial comparisons administered about every six weeks will help for evaluation purposes. Most patients will show a measurable decrease in Resting HR and submaximal work level HR from their pre-training test to their six-week test.

CARDIAC REHABILITATION AND HEART RATE MONITORING: PHASE III PROGRAMS...AND BEYOND

Phase III programs are extended, supervised, outpatient programs which include patients who are 6–12 weeks post-hospital discharge, have clinically stable or decreasing symptoms and the ability to self-regulate their exercise. These Phase III participants rely on follow-up exercise testing and medical evaluation based on their primary physician's recommendations. This regular medical follow-up is essential on a three to six month basis and eventually on an annual basis or as needed.

Exercise prescriptions for Phase III should be gradually increased up to a duration of 45 minutes or more, to an intensity of 50–85% of functional capacity, three to five days per week. Functional capacity is based on the patient's clinical status and pathological abnormalities and is usually measured in ability to sustain workload (measured in METs).

The primary goal of Phase III is to promote adherence to the exercise prescription and other behavior modification goals to the point where the patient is a lifelong exercise participant. One of the values of using a heart rate monitor in an exercise program is the motivational factor that it provides; it is a key ingredient to sustaining lifelong participation.

One question that many cardiac patients raise, not surprisingly, is about sex. When can they return to their normal sexual activity? There are psychological fears that a myocardial infarction (heart attack) and medications such as beta-blocking agents and diuretics can cause sexual impairment. It is unclear from the research to date whether cardiac rehabilitation programs, specifically exercise, have a positive impact on sexual function, including interest and desire. Adequate counseling in the form of education and referrals to specialists are an essential part of cardiac rehabilitation efforts.

In many ways, sexual activity is a form of exercise. Sex burns about the same number of calories on the average as walking up three flights of stairs. The average heart rate range during sexual intercourse is between 115–120 bpm, and at the peak (during orgasm), the heart rate can rise above 120 bpm.

Even with a reduction in the postcoronary patient's aerobic capacity, over 80% of them can still perform without symptoms both sexually and in the majority of jobs that require low physical work demands. Because of sexual activity's brief duration, the low frequency in middle-aged and older individuals, the modest heart rate and oxygen demands (not to mention the patient's general happiness), most heart doctors encourage their patients to resume sexual activity.

Heart rate monitors can reassure the cardiac rehabilitation patient that they are exercising at a safe, productive intensity level. There should never be a fear of exercise if it is well monitored and planned. The only fear you should have is a fear of inactivity. A well thought out training program keeps you on track for a healthier, positive, active lifestyle. Not only will you live longer, you'll enjoy it more along the way as well.

AFTER A QUADRUPLE BYPASS, THE HEART RATE MONITOR
THE STORY OF ALBERT HARDAKER

The story of Albert Hardaker: Everybody at the Court House Racquet Club in Florence, Alabama, knows Albert "Tink" Hardaker, and he jokingly refers to himself as an unpaid assistant instructor. The reason for the 64 year-old's popularity is that he spends six mornings a week at the center, working out and assisting unofficially in the senior citizen classes.

Tink Hardaker arrived at the Club two years ago, looking for help in rehabilitating from quadruple bypass heart surgery and the addition of a pacemaker. After discharge from the hospital, he had been told to "walk," but was not given instructions as to distances or speeds. He decided to join the Racquet Club and entered the Seniors Aerobics Class where, for the first time in his life, he began a regular workout routine.

Hardaker noticed the Club's wireless heart rate monitor and asked to try it out. He was taken with the monitor, especially its target heart zone feature, and he was quick to purchase his own. It wasn't long before Tink devised his own 30 minute, 140 bpm, treadmill workout, which is now an essential part of his daily regimen. On days when he needs a rest from this pace, he'll walk at 120 bpm.

Tink says his current lifestyle has made him feel physically and mentally better than at any time he can remember. And the reputation he's acquired among the Club's members is a great bonus.

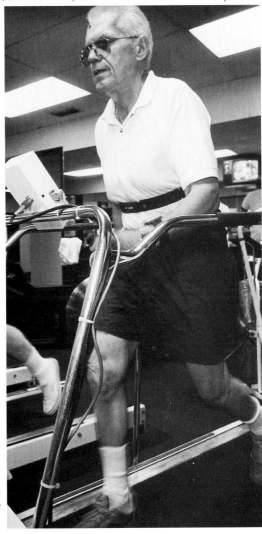

Tink Hardaker, quadruple bypass survivor, athlete and local hero.

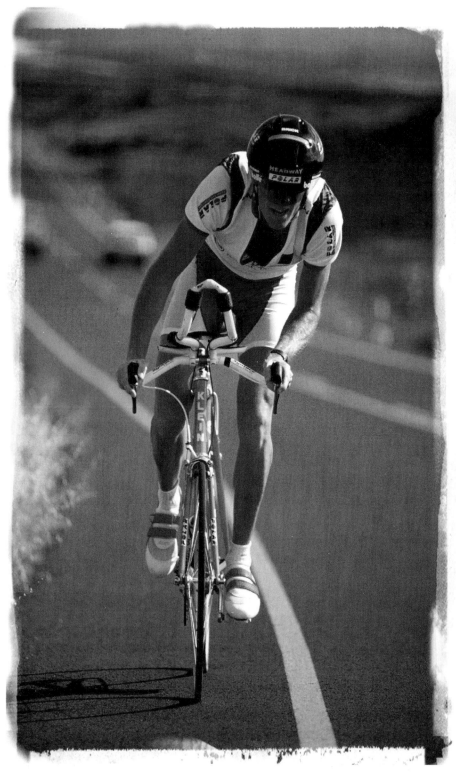

CHAPTER TWELVE

HIGH
PERFORMANCE

The quest for higher levels of human performance has been going on for a long time. Maybe the drive to excel is a leftover from a time when there were two choices: perform or die. Of course, that was a long time ago. We no longer have to worry about chasing fleet-footed animals across rolling plains, hooting and hollering under a blue, smog-free sky (sounds fun doesn't it?).

ow, most of us hop around the corner to the local store if we're hungry. Sometimes when I get home, I hold a bunch of broccoli over my head and let out a triumphant shout; the great huntress returns with her kill. But it's just not the same. Vegetarians sometimes do get left out of certain traditions.

Now, that prehistoric drive remains largely unchanged and untapped, but it can be pulled out of even the most sedentary of beings with a little effort. Sports scientists, including physiologists, nutritionists, biochemists, and psychologists, focus on assisting athletes towards honing that drive, towards achieving higher and higher goals. What athletes strive so hard for these days is their optimal training intensity, which is directly correlated with their anaerobic threshold level (AT).

ANAEROBIC THRESHOLD TRAINING

If the term "anaerobic threshold" (AT) is not yet quite clear to you, there is a reason; AT has been associated with such a wide range of terms and ideas (respiratory exchange ratios, blood lactate concentrations, oxygen utilization measurements, and heart rate responses to name a few) that few athletes are clear on exactly what an anaerobic threshold really is.

A quick biochemical and practical explanation of lactates might help you understand AT better. The point when your muscles are beginning to ache and burn from fatigue is not the point when your body is just beginning to produce lactic acid, but is instead the point when your body can no longer immediately get rid of it. So this point, the AT, is the intensity level at which the body produces more lactic acid (the by-product of muscle contractions) than it can eliminate. AT is also called lactic turnpoint, lactate threshold, OBLA (onset of blood lactate accumulation) or heart rate breakpoint. It is the break-even point of exercise effort, where there is just enough oxygen and just enough lactic acid for the two to stay in balance. It also follows that as workout intensity increases, so do blood lactate concentrations.

Now obviously it would be a very good thing to be able to exercise harder and not get further and further dragged down by the pains of lactate accumulation. This is where AT training (at 80%–90% of your Max HR) comes in. The purpose of AT training is to teach your metabolic system to clear lactates out of your muscles more efficiently. According to Dr. George Brooks, Director of Exercise Physiology at the University of California at Berkeley, the rate of an individual's lactate clearance can improve one hundred percent with training. That is something worth shooting for.

All this being said, determining AT levels, (whether on the basis of a mathematical equation or by blood lactate testing) is important to athletes, because it remains the best method of predicting endurance performance. Experienced athletes generally race at intensity levels near or slightly above their AT point, rather than their Max VO2 point, thus workout intensity at the AT point is considered to be the most powerful and consistent predictor of aerobic exercise capability today.

Here are the AT training rules of thumb:

• The closer you can train to your AT, the more your AT level increases.

• Like Max HR levels, your AT is sport-specific. This specificity is probably the result of variations in the mass and fitness of the different muscle masses activated.

• The closer your AT level gets to your Max HR, the better your performance.

• Workouts far below AT intensity are ineffective in raising your performance level.

• Too many workouts above your AT are also ineffective, due to the effects of overtraining.

• The best and fastest marathon pace is slightly slower than your AT pace.

• The best and fastest 10k pace is typically faster than your AT pace.

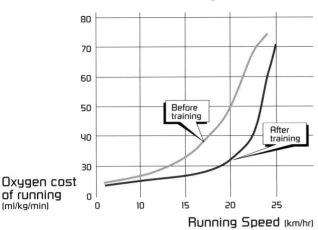

The Anaerobic Training Effect

Oxygen cost of running (ml/kg/min)

Running Speed (km/hr)

Before training

After training

HEART RATE LEVELS AND ANAEROBIC THRESHOLD:
THE CONCONI TEST

An Italian biochemical researcher at the University of Ferrara, Italy, Dr. Francesco Conconi is solely credited for equating heart rate levels with AT levels. Basically, Conconi's research lead him to the determination that at some point, the heart rate becomes incapable of increasing in linear fashion with exercise intensity. This point is called the heart rate deflection point (we call it the AT), and the speed of the athlete at that point is called the deflection velocity. The deflection point is one of the best predictors of performance available today. However, not all athletes have a specific deflection point; for some athletes a deflection point can be determined from the deflection curve.

The Conconi Test (or AT Test, as we call it today) is a very simple, non-invasive method of determining your current heart rate level at its anaerobic threshold point. There are other methods for determining AT, but they require drawing blood samples during exercise or using complex medical equipment to detect alterations in your respiratory gases.

Using his test, Conconi devised a training program using periodic workouts at heart rates close to threshold for Francesco Moser, then a 33 year-old cyclist and the 1977 world professional road champion. Conconi used anaerobic threshold training as the cornerstone of Moser's special training program, and the result astonished the cycling community as Moser broke the World Hour Record twice in January, 1984. Many attributed Moser's success to technological advantages: carbon fiber wheels, altitude, the computerized monitoring of Moser's average and ideal speeds, the faster track surface, a special bike, and an aerodynamic bodysuit. But in fact, it wasn't the equipment or the environment which propelled Moser to victory. It was the physiological changes in Moser that had been produced by Conconi's heart rate monitor training program. Simply put, Moser trained magnificently.

Now, Conconi's findings are not bullet-proof. David Martin, Professor of Health Sciences at Georgia State University and chairperson of TAC's Sport Sciences, states, "There is no logical reason for the heart to have a deflection point; there is no logical reason for the relationship to be anything but linear."

Martin adds, "Conconi indeed found in all of his 210 runners that as the heart rate rose with an increasing workload, there was a point where the linear rate of rise changed to a new rate. But when he studied a subset of 26 of these to identify whether this change occurred at the AT, it did in only 10. That's less than half the runner population—hardly common enough to warrant its general use in testing and training. Other workers trying to duplicate his studies have had similar lack of success; some do not see a departure from linearity at all." In fact, quite frequently world class female athletes find that their AT pace heart rate is the same as their maximum heart rate, with no deflections in the rate of the rise of their heart rate or lactates. So, take Conconi with a grain of salt, but take him if you like.

Martin, on the other hand, recommends the "2 x 20 Minute Anaerobic Threshold Test." This AT test calls for a long, sustained effort that is faster than your low intensity Sunday run but slower than your red-line pace. To do the test, complete two 20 minute intervals of your favored sport activity. Keep track of your heart rate at each one minute interval, as well as your finish time. After completing both 20 minute intervals, answer the question: was that the hardest that I could run (ski, bike, swim) for that duration of time (40 minutes total)? If the answer is yes, then that heart rate/pace is within a 5 bpm range of your AT training pace and AT heart rate.

There is definitely some degree of question among research sports scientists about the entire concept of anaerobic threshold as a specific deflection point. Many contend that since lactate accumulates throughout all workouts at all intensity levels, there is no actual "point" but rather an anaerobic zone, a range of heart rates at which the lactate accumulation curve, relative to training intensity, becomes greater than a 10 degree slope (this is calculated mathematically by determining the slope or steepness on a graph). For most purposes though, it is probably fine to just determine your anaerobic zone as we did a few chapters back, as 80% to 90% of your Max HR.

HEART RATE DRIFT

One of the reasons I love to use my heart rate monitor is because it's fun—it is my favorite toy. One of my favorite games I play with my heart rate monitor is "How High, How Fast"—how high will my heart rate get, depending on how fast I go.

The first time I played the game I was riding the White Bullet (a Kestrel 4000 racing bike) and simultaneously turned on my cyclometer and my heart rate monitor. I watched the two electronic gadgets in play with one another as I learned how my heart responded to my exertions. I started at 140 bpm and 16 mph, my steady-state warm-up speed. I then decided to see how many bpm each mph on the bike would cost. The results surprised me.

For every one mph of increased bike speed, my heart rate increased exponentially. At 17 mph my heart rate rose to 145. Riding at 18 mph it rose to 151. At 19 mph my heart rate was 158. Riding at 20 mph my bpm was at 166 beats, and at 21 mph it went to 175 beats, but at 22 mph the exertion cost me 185 bpm. At that point, I said "whoa" to the White Bullet and dropped back down to a more comfortable 170 bpm. I kept my heart rate steady the rest of the ride and had one of my fastest bike times ever.

Now, aside from examples of sheer bravado like that above, there is another important reason why your heart rate may increase significantly over the course of a training session. That reason is heart rate drift, also known as "cardiac drift," and it is the gradual increase in heart rate during long workouts due to the prolonged effects of fatigue, increased body temperature, and likely dehydration. Physiologically speaking, the heart works to provide a sufficient amount of cardiac output to sustain the workload, keeping the amount of blood that is delivered to muscles in balance with the demand. To do this, as you exercise harder and your muscles demand more freshly oxygenated blood, the heart must either increase its number of beats per minute or the amount of blood it pumps with each beat (stroke volume).

This is where cardiac drift comes into play. As you exercise, the heart is forced to increase the number of bpm, because it is compensating for a decreasing stroke volume caused by losses in plasma volume. In hot weather, cardiac drift is more prevalent because of dehydration. The opposite is also true in colder weather, where there is less cardiac drift, because the body does not perspire as much and hence loses less blood volume.

Look at the print-out below and notice the heart rate drift. The athlete is not increasing her speed or intensity, but her heart rate is being forced to accommodate decreased stroke volume by slowly raising its cardiac frequency.

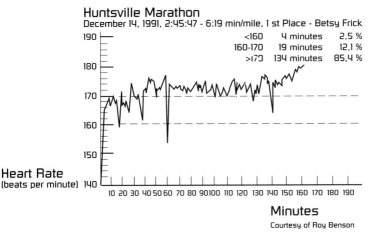

When we first started racing and training with heart rate monitors (this was in 1984), my training partner Karen Coe and I had a classic starting line disagreement: would we race by pace or heart rate. At the beginning of the Pepsi 20 Miler in Clarksburg, California, she wanted start and finish at a 6:45-

7:00 min/mile pace, and I wanted to race at a 160 bpm pace. We were both training to qualify for the USA Olympic Marathon Trials, and the race was a key training workout for us.

The argument wasn't settled when the starting gun sent us off, and we continued the debate until we hit the one mile marker. The mile split was 6:45, and our heart rates were within one to two beats of one another at 160 bpm. What was more interesting to me, though, was that I got to watch cardiac drift in action. At mile 10, pace 6:45, our heart rates were at about 160. At mile 15, pace 6:45, we were at 168 bpm. With each mile, pace maintained, our heart rates floated ever higher. At mile 19 we were soaring at a pace of 6:45 and a heart rate of 180. We agreed to really kick it in for the last mile. It seemed like we were flying over our last mile split, but we weren't. As we gave it all we got, we were only getting a minimal increase in pace (6:30), for a big jump in heart rate (190 bpm).

We were thrilled at the end of the race. To have that kind of reliable biofeedback during a race fascinated me. I have raced with a heart rate monitor ever since, and I am always careful to note my cardiac drift. Making adjustments for the drift, and keeping a close eye on my heart rate monitor has helped me through enough races and training runs to fill this book and another like it.

And yes, later that same year, I qualified for the first ever women's Olympic Marathon Trials.

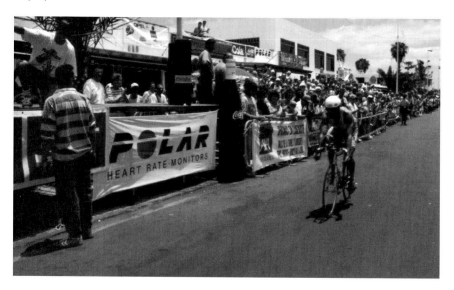

RACING TIPS WITH A HEART RATE MONITOR

After ten years of racing with a heart rate monitor, I have learned just how valuable my coach, the heart rate monitor, can be for me. When I race with it and then download the data into my personal computer afterwards, I can relive the experience and it reveals real truths: did I pace evenly, did I go out too fast, was my warm-up before the race sufficient, am I overtrained.

But most of all, I use the heart rate monitor for pacing. If you can find out your "heart rate AT" that is your heart rate number when you reach the AT point, then all you have to do is factor in the distance of the race and calculate a racing heart rate. Here's my basic rule.

Short Races (under one hour in lenght): heart rate 3-5 bpm over AT

Intermediate Distance Races (one hour): heart rate at AT

Long Distance Races (marathon and over 40K bike time trials): heart rate 3-5 bpm under AT.

Your AT level changes with conditioning. When I am in great shape, my AT is 90-92% of my Max HR. Also remember that AT like Max HR is sport specific. Usually cycling AT heart rates are 5-10 bpm lower than running and swimming another 5-10 bpm lower than cycling. For multi-sport racing athletes, one of the goals is to close this AT threshold difference. Matt Brick, a champion duathlete, has been able to squeeze his two different AT's -- cycling AT and running AT -- to within 2-3 beats of each other. That's a sign of well-balanced and well-training multi-sport athlete.

DIAGNOSING TRAINING WITH A HEART RATE MONITOR

After your heart rate monitor becomes a part of your regular training, you can even fine tune your workouts by allowing the information that it provides to show you the way. In this way, your heart rate monitor becomes a way for you to self-diagnose if you are feeling that there are problems but are uncertain as to them.

Here are a few quick pointers that might help you stay training longer and happier because you are heeding to the link between the mind and the body -- the heart rate monitor:

Condition: The Sluggish Heart Rate. If you notice that when you add intensity like climbing a hill, your heart rate is slow to respond and when you have reached the top it is slower than normal in recovery, then listen to your heart.
Diagnosis: Probably, you are overtrained or tired.
Response: Reduce your training volume with no interval training until condition disappears.
Condition: The Self-Test for Over conditioning. This is an easy test that you can administer to yourself at almost anywhere and anytime. Lie flat for several minutes and rest. Take your heart rate. Stand up. Take your heart rate. If there is a 20 beat or bigger difference then take note.
Diagnosis: Probably, you are overtrained or tired.
Response: Rest.
Condition: Heart Rate Drift. In this situation, you are training at an even pace and the environmental conditions are unchanged. Slowly, you notice that your heart rate is increasing without an increase in the exercise intensity.
Diagnosis: Dehydration and decrease in blood volume.
Response: Drink fluids immediately and in the future based on time not feeling.

Condition:Heart Rate Drop. As you are working out you note that the opposite happens, your heart rate is dropping but you think you are maintaining the same intensity.

Diagnosis: Could be "the bonk" or "the wall". You probably have not eaten enough of the right calories or you have not training your endurance training systems enough to handle the workout.

Response: Eat. Or, train more gradually and work your way up by practicing long slow distance training. Or, rest.

Condition: AT Unreachable. This happens during interval workouts and you just can´t get your heart rate high enough to reach you AT heart rate.

Diagnosis: Probably, you are overtrained or tired.

Response: Stop interval training for awhile and rest or do recovery workouts.

Condition: High Heart Rate. It feels easy and comfortable and yet your monitor is telling you that you are working out at very high training zones.

Diagnosis: One of the following: upcoming illness (cold, flu, viral infection is around the bend), it´s early in the season, not recovered from previous workouts or probably, you are overtrained or tired.

Response: Rest.

INTERVAL TRAINING WITH A HEART RATE MONITOR

If you want to race fast, train fast. But even though increasing your speed in miles per hour is about as positive an addiction as I know, it's not the most efficient way to train. Don't train by how fast your body is moving through space, train by how fast your heart is beating inside you.

There are a number of excellent high intensity/interval workouts in the anaerobic threshold and red-line sections of chapter 6 and throughout this book in the "From Experience" sections at the end of most chapters. Try them out. As you design your training program and write it into your Heart Rate Monitor Planner Log, set down your high and low heart rate limits for the interval workout. Following are examples of typical speed intervals: run at 180-185 bpm 2 x 1 miles (two one-mile intervals) and 3 x 3/4 mile (three three-quarter mile intervals). Look at the following interval. Can you tell what's wrong with it?

Running Interval
Sally Edwards 6 / 15 / 92; 2 x 1 mile and 3 x 3/4 mile, with a rest interval of 1/4 mile jog

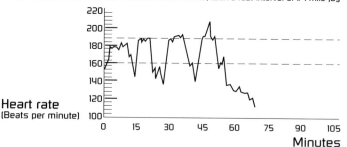

Heart rate
(Beats per minute)

Analyzing your heart rate workouts, such as the one above, is key to your understanding program design (the real secret weapon in training). Heart rate monitors should not be used as speedometers or better still odometers—they are really planning tools. The problem with the interval workout above was that my plan had called for 180–185 bpm for all five intervals, but the fourth interval was at 195-200 bpm. I pushed myself too hard, crashed and quit the workout never finishing the fifth interval.

There are a number of high performance athletes who have not yet tried to use a heart rate monitor. You may be one of those, reading this book looking for the secret weapon or the smoking gun. According to George Parrott, Sacramento State University professor and running coach, "The reasons I think that my best runners don't use one are the following, in descending order: unwillingness to go to the edge, fears of failure or success, denial in the hope they won't have to train with intensity or concern that they might have to slow down and use them like brakes."

Others think they don't need a heart rate monitor because they can manually take their pulse rate instead. Beware. In some individuals, strong pressure from your fingers against your carotid artery (on your neck) may produce an immediate reaction—the heart rate slows. If you are one of these individuals, counting your pulse rate may give you numbers that are consistently too low, causing you to train higher than the target heart rate zone you have selected. To check to see if you are getting falsely low readings, change methods and compare the results. Either take your pulse at your radial artery (on your wrist), which causes no change in heart rates or, better yet, use a heart rate monitor.

Ultimately, training is a blend of art and of science. The heart rate monitor is the science in the blend, and you provide the creative part that leads to a high quality, fine-tuned individualized program. No piece of equipment will ever take that away from you.

It is unlikely our ancient ancestors sat around their cave fires and worried about lactic acid build-up or anaerobic thresholds. Seldom were any of them seen limping after a fleeing elk, holding their legs and screaming, "Owww, oww, my lactate production seems to have exceeded my local rate of lactate consumption...owwww!" They knew only one thing: perform or die

We've come a long way since then. You can now go down to a track and witness athletes running around in circles screaming, "Owww, oww, my lactate production seems to have exceeded my local rate of lactate consumption...owwww!" But the hunt now is for an elusive yet attainable reward. That reward is a mental one; it lies deep in the psyche of athletes, and it drives them to personal bests, world records, and feats at which others can only marvel. The tools that enabled the ancient hunter to survive—guile, speed, intelligence—are exactly the tools you need to push your own performance to higher levels. Learn your AT and your optimum training levels and train with guile, intelligence, and consistency; these will give you speed. Our ancestors would be proud.

Basic Rules

Here are some basic training rules that you need to know and follow in all five intensities of heart rate monitored workouts.

1. **48-HOUR RULE:** After an aerobic or red-line workout, the body requires 48 hours of rest and/or exercise at a lower intensity level, before it can again be treated to another dose of anaerobic or red-line intensity in the same sports activity.

2. **24-HOUR RULE:** If you cross-train, only one anaerobic or red-line workout in a different sport activity in each 24 hour period.

3. **TRAIN SPARINGLY AT YOUR UPPER LIMITS.** Don't train regularly at the red-line heart level. If you do, not only will you suffer, you will probably be on track for an injury.

4. **THE 10% AND 25% RULES.** A single anaerobic or red-line workout should not be greater than 10% of your weekly mileage. The sum of all anaerobic or red-line workouts should not exceed 25% of your total weekly mileage.

WORKOUTS FOR ULTRA-DISTANCE ATHLETES

As an ultra-distance triathlon specialist, I have found the use of heart rate monitors to be essential to the success of my training program. Each of my training sessions has a specific objective and my heart rate monitor allows me to match this objective closely.

I've found that heart rate monitors also aid in the development of two key skills for the athlete. The first is matching heart rate with perceived exertion, the feeling of effort. By using a heart rate monitor you learn to associate what specific intensities or paces feel like and can use this in races to guide your performance. Second, I have found that the heart rate monitor is a useful tool to signal overtraining or lack of recovery from racing or training. In my experience the heart rate/perceived exertion relationship breaks down when I am not fully recovered, causing a high level of perceived exertion to correspond to a low heart rate. For example, during a cycling interval session my heart rate should be between 165 and 175 bpm and the effort should feel hard. If I am not recovered or am overtrained, the same feeling corresponds to a heart rate of 145-155 bpm. If this happens at the beginning of a training session, I turn around and go home to rest.

I use my heart rate monitor for almost all of my workouts (except for very easy recovery sessions), but I have found a couple of situations where they are particularly useful. The first is in LSD (long, slow distance) cycling and running workouts. The objective of these sessions is to keep the intensity low (65% max HR) and the duration long (5+ hours cycling, 2+ hours running).

The monitor helps me to do three things during these workouts. First, the heart rate monitor is essential to my keeping the intensity low enough, especially going uphill. Second, the heart rate monitor allows me to keep the intensity high enough on downhills. Instead of just cruising on the downhills, I try to keep my heart rate in the proper range by spinning down the hills on the bike and lengthening my stride when running. This helps me develop a keen sense of effort on all types of terrain. Third, my heart rate monitor allows me to control the pace in a group situation, so I can still meet the objective of my workout. Most group situations tend to get less social as the session goes on, and as a result, the pace increases. By using my heart rate monitor as a pacing guide, I can control my effort and let the group go ahead if they start to hammer, or I can find people with whom I can do these sessions and still stay in control.

In addition to LSD sessions, another of my favorite types of training with a heart rate monitor is long, steady, race pace efforts on the bike. I usually do a 2–3 hour time trial at the Ironman distance race pace (24–25 mph) once every 2 weeks. The intensity is moderately high, but it is certainly sustainable, about 80–85% of my maximum heart rate. The goal here is to become more efficient and focused during a long effort, and I try to keep the pace where I want it and lower my heart rate at the same time. This forces me to experiment with technique to find the most efficient cadence and pedaling style, as well as working on focusing techniques. I find that if I focus on my breathing and biomechanics, I can ride at the same pace with a lower heart rate. These types of sessions also help me to evaluate my fitness and make changes in my program to match my fitness level, something we all should do every 6–8 weeks.

Ray Browning is a seven-time Ironman Triathlon Champion.

The HISTORY

O F   T H E   H E A R T   R A T E   M O N I T O R

I think it's important to trace the progress of heart rate monitors from their beginnings as a training tool through their development into a product for the general public. History can lend great insight into the present, and so it is with heart rate monitors.

The best place to start is at the beginning. Imagine early cave dwellers, lying quietly at night, feeling the pulse of their heart in their veins. They must have been aware of the heart's rhythms, aware of the most consistent beat they had ever heard. Surely, one of the cave dwellers palpated an artery and noticed their pulse. They might not have known what it was, but I doubt they thought it trivial.

Chinese healers have for millennia used what they called the "three finger method" to diagnose their patients. They would place three of their fingers over their patients' wrists to detect both blood pressure and pulse rate. They realized many centuries ago that this information could be used to diagnose illnesses.

The idea for modern day heart rate monitors came about one day during a training workout. Seppo Saynajakangas, a professor of electronics at Oulu University in Finland, went skiing with a friend who happened to be a Nordic ski coach. The coach, knowing Seppo's background, asked for a way to reliably measure the heart rate of his Nordic skiers. What was important, thought the coach, was to know his racers' training heart rates for conditioning purposes and to use their heart rates as a kind of index scale for fitness.

This request inspired Seppo. He researched what was available and found that photo-reflectance units such as ear clip or finger tip pulse monitors

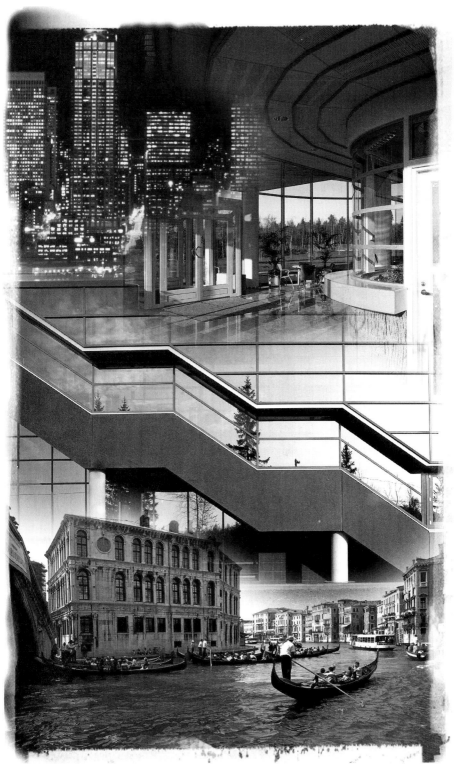

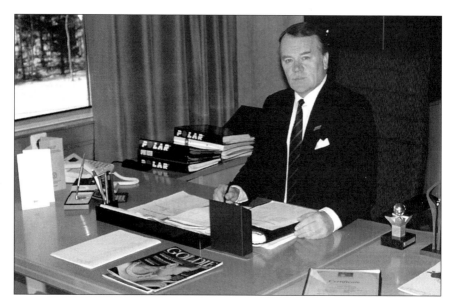

Dr. Seppo Säynäjäkangas, the inventor of wireless heart rate monitors.

were neither reliable for athletes who were strenuously exerting themselves or handy, because of the wires involved. He decided that the existing electrocardiograph (ECG) monitors which measured the heart's electrical activity were the way to go, but they were too bulky and expensive for personal use. His solution was to translate the ECG technology into a portable form, and he developed his own mathematical algorithms to do so. In his quest to develop the methodology of wireless transmission of electrical heart rate signals, Dr. Säynäjäkangas requested and received research support from The Finnish Academy and the Finnish Olympic Committee. After enough data had been collected and the early prototypes designed and tested, it became clear that a viable commercial product could be developed from the research ideas that were being grown in the Electronics Laboratory at Oulu University.

Seppo Säynäjäkangas founded Polar Electro Oy in 1977 as a company that would continue the research and development of commercial heart rate monitors and eventually manufacture the first wireless heart rate monitors. It took five years of research and development to bring his first commercial heart monitors to market, but he did. In 1982 Seppo Säynäjäkangas filed and received the first worldwide patents on the product—wireless, short distance ECG telemetry heart rate monitors.

There were others in the early days of scientific sports training that knew that there was a relationship between heart rate training and performance success. The former East Germany's cycling coach, Wolfram Lindner (today considered "the father" of German cycling) was one of the first to employ heart rate training methods and with significant success.

In the mid-1970s, Lindner and Dr. Dietmar Junkar, exercise science professor at the University of Leipzig, built a transmitter belt that he attached to the cyclists' clothing. The belt used a radio antenna that transmitted to a receiver in a car following the riders. Coaches would listen to the heart rate through earphones and count the beats that they heard and record them. This was a painstaking, laborious system of listening for hours to heart beats, which were then manually transferred to graph paper to serve as a record of the training session. It may have been horribly dull work, but it paid off. Their team became a world cycling powerhouse.

In 1982 Polar Electro Oy introduced the world to the first wireless heart rate monitors. These first generation heart rate monitors (the "PE 2000s") were released onto the market and readily accepted by athletes, particularly at the elite and national levels. The PE 2000 was immediately accepted and sold in over 20 countries around the world. Athletes and trainers still continued to jot down heart rate values by hand, however, until 1984 when Polar Electro Oy developed the key software and interface system that stored the heart rate data for later computer downloading and analysis.

By December 1984, the second generation of wireless heart rate monitors called PE 3000 by Polar, but marketed as the Quantum XL, Uniq CIC Heartwatch, and the Sport Tester 3000, were released with computer interface equipment and software. Polar allowed other companies to put their name on the PE 3000 in a private label agreement so they could continue to focus on research and development, leaving the marketing and education surrounding the product to more established companies in the fitness equipment industry.

Polar knew then that the recreational heart rate monitor user market was both tremendous and untapped. By 1987, they had developed additional models with fewer features, which cut their retail price and made the heart rate monitor much more available to the recreational athlete. The PE 300 (commercially named the Uniq CIC ProTrainer or Sport Tester PE 300) allowed the common athlete easy access to what was previously "high performance athlete only" equipment.

Meanwhile, more companies entered the market. In 1985, Nike introduced a device which used ECG technology and a black box strapped around the waist that served as a receiver. Designed by Ned Frederick and his staff, the model featured a computer-generated voice that read out heart rate, distance travelled, and elapsed time through headphones. There was no monitor or visual display. Nike dissolved the division that produced the heart rate monitors after they failed to sell, and a half-dozen other companies that had launched products around the same time also met a similar demise. In 1987 several Japanese companies, including Sanyo, also introduced heart rate monitors, but as their technology was copied from Polar, their products did not have much of an impact in the history of monitors' ongoing technological development.

The year 1990 heralded the arrival of a full product line for Polar with the release of the Vantage XL or Sport Tester models which were enhanced models of the PE 3000. The company also released the Accurex, Pacer, Cyclovantage, and Optimex. Likewise, they decided to unify their business by marketing and distributing their products solely under their own brand name, Polar, discontinuing all of their private label business.

Polar's largest distributor of it´s wireless heart rate monitors was Computer Instruments Corporation (CIC) in New York. The American company had taken a slightly different track in the search for a training heart monitor; starting with Burt Birnbaum's development of the first fingertip pulsemeters in 1973, CIC had a long tradition as the leading manufacturer and distributor of pulsemeters in the world. From 1987 to 1991, CIC was also the exclusive distributor of Polar's products.

With the American company CIC leading the way, the pulsemeter market grew as they were marketed to the general consumer concerned with health and fitness. Meanwhile, the Polar Electro Oy company in Finland was expanding the heart rate monitor market. Asian companies on the other hand were trying to copy the technology from both and duplicate their products at a price point that would attract business to them. Most of these secondary ventures lead to failure, simply because the technology behind heart rate monitors and pulsemeters was continuing to develop at an ever-increasing rate that the upstart companies could not keep up with. Also, Polar's proprietary grip was firmly in place.

In 1991, Casio entered the market for the first time with their BP 100, a photo-reflectance unit that measures both blood pressure and pulse rate. The unit requires that the user hold completley still for it to provide accurate data—hardly a realistic option for most people.

At the end of 1991 Polar Electro, the parent company of Polar USA, Inc., purchased the health and fitness division of their USA distributor, Computer Instruments Corporation (CIC), and the two companies combined into one: Polar CIC. Simultaneously, Polar Electro Oy released many new, highly affordable models such as the Edge and Favor, the distribution of which is taken care of by Polar CIC in the United States.

The greatest advances in heart rate monitors for the rest of this decade should be in three areas where there already has been great advancement: cost, memory and technology due to the continuous breakthroughs in computer microchip technology.

A PERSONAL HISTORY OF HEART RATE MONITOR TRAINING

My association with the field of sports medicine began in 1981 when I finished medical school and wrote my thesis on professional bicyclists. I went on to become the director of the Italian Research Center for Sport and Preventive Medicine; there athletes are tested to see if they can pass the extensive medical examination necessary for them (by law!) to compete professionally in Italy, and of course, heart rate monitors have become one of the central tools to do the testing.

As a medical doctor, from my point of view, heart rate

monitors are central to all aspects of sports medicine: testing, rehabilitation, and training. When I started in my field, wireless heart rate monitors were not available for our use, so we had to make due with clumsier equipment and less complete results. For example, bicyclists could not perform indoors, strung up with wires, as they normally would in a race. Thanks to wireless heart rate monitors, everything is easier, and the memory storage capabilities which allow us to download information after it is recorded out on the course, have been most valuable to our research.

I have worked with Polar for many years; they are the official supplier of heart rate monitors for the Research Center's studies. We once had over 300 coaches at our facility who spent two days learning about heart rate monitors and the attached exercise equipment; these tools are considered key to Italy's training programs.

In 1985 I began attending races and working out in the field with what is now the Motorola Cycling Team (it used to be the 7-11 team). Now during the Tour de France I take a portable computer, the Polar software, and heart rate monitors, so that I can monitor the members of our team. The athletes wear the chest belts every day and say they are comfortable during the entire race. Using heart rate monitors has allowed us to determine that the cyclists' heart rate profiles are not at all the same at the beginning of the tour as at the end. The riders can reach their maximum heart rates easily at the beginning of the first week of the race, but by the end of the tour, due to the increasing effects of fatigue, their maximum heart rates can be up to 10 bpm less. In planning training and racing strategies, we have found that it is much more important at any given time to know how fast the cyclists' hearts are going than to know the speed of their bicycles.

We also do rehabilitation for heart attack and heart bypass surgery patients at the Research Center. We monitor the patients' exertion with heart rate monitors, and we always know when they are exercising within the limits we have set, due to the programmable alarms on the monitors. The patients, too, feel more secure this way, since they know how hard their hearts are working at any time and are alerted whenever they might be overexerting.

In addition to athletes and rehabilitators, there are also many people who benefit from using heart rate monitors to lose weight, but I have even found monitors useful in helping those who have trouble keeping weight on. Through extensive testing using heart rate monitors and other equipment, we determined the metabolic costs of the exercise routines of a group of ballet dancers in Milan who were losing weight. Once we brought their diet in line with their metabolic needs, they were fine.

I am delighted to be part of this field at a time when such marvelous technology is available. Heart rate monitors have spoiled all of us, athlete and researcher, very much.

Dr. Massimo Testa's long history in the sports medicine field is currently highlighted by his positions as Team Physician for the world-class Motorola Cycling Team and Director of the Italian Research Center for Sport and Preventive Medicine.

LIVE A LONGER AND HAPPIER LIFE

Heart rate monitors provide the link between the body's physical intensity and the mind's need for data. They provide the tangible proof of progress that encourages you to work out more diligently and safely. They are powerful physical and psychological tools.

I f you were one of those who were so initially confounded by heart rate monitors that yours has been gathering dust, rest assured that you have not been alone in your frustration. You and others like you are why I wrote this book; never before have I been so impressed after being so frustrated with a training tool.

What I finally learned with the help of my heart rate monitor is that fitness is about heart rate, not pace. To optimize the limited amount of time that we all have to get in shape, it is absolutely more effective to measure how hard we are exerting ourselves by using heart rate monitors, rather than to just try to hit pacing goals on our exercise bikes or rowing machines. By nature, pace charts are not particularly individualized things, but heart rates and heart rate monitors are, which is what makes heart rate monitors so very nice. For example, if you are fit, your Resting HR will be low and your training program will be of higher intensity. On the flip side, if you are unfit, your Resting HR will be high and your training program will only need to be of a lower intensity to achieve your proper training heart rate. In either case, your heart rate monitor will be your faithful guide and companion.

After all of the tests I've been through as an athlete, let me tell you something that I hope you'll never have to find out for yourselves: it can hurt to measure fitness. Over the years I have been prodded, taped, strapped,

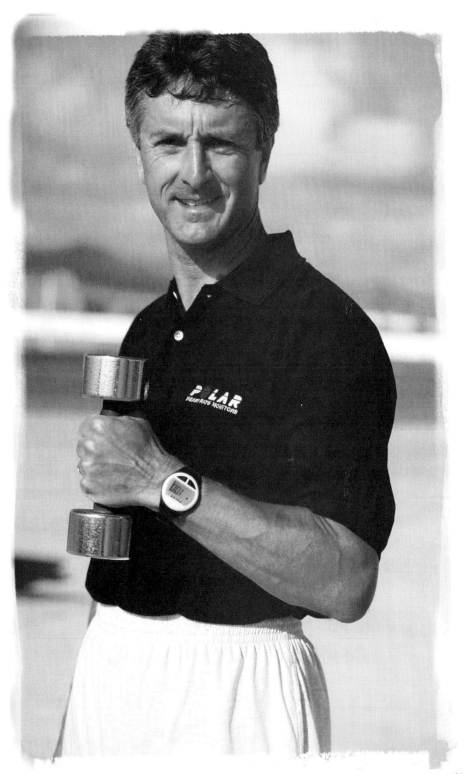

pricked, put on treadmills and run into the ground to get the kind of information heart rate monitors beep out painlessly.

Finally, for me, a heart rate monitor is more than a gadget or a fitness tool. It is a way to reach my ultimate individual life goal. Sound dramatic? Let me explain.

For the past half dozen years I have both trained and raced regularly with a heart rate monitor. It has been one of those essential "secrets" that I tell everyone about and that has kept me competing for so many years without major down time. I have purchased four or five different models and found some that work really well and others that quite frankly don't. And, as they have improved, so have I. I have not become a slave to heart rate monitors—I don't feel naked or blind when I don't wear one—because my heart rate monitors have helped me to learn to know my heart rates as well as my training course's rocks and curves.

At the 1991 Ironman Triathlon, I was racing to win the master's (40–44 years) age division. As always, I set my race plan and visualized it in advance. On race day I replayed that mental video. I knew just about when the monkey of fatigue was going to jump on my back during the 112 mile bike leg. I knew when the triathlon hammer was going to first pound on my legs and then lock-em-up after the bike-to-run transition. I knew what inner strength it would take to dig into my deep down confidence to run the 26.2 mile marathon at 172 beats per minute.

This was to be my 13th Ironman distance race. I knew the split times and the course conditions, the heat and humidity, black lava fields and tough competition, and I knew myself and my conditioning level.

The race went almost exactly as planned. The swim split was exact to my time calculations, so I took off on my Specialized Allez carbon fiber bike and settled into the bike leg heart rate plan: 155–160 regardless of the number of cyclists who wanted to race faster or harder (they flew by me in the early stages). I knew I would catch them later.

When I dismounted the Allez, the triathlon had already taken a toll on my quads. I took the heart rate monitor off my handlebars and strapped it around my wrist. I slipped on a pair of Nike Air Mariahs and took off at my run pulse (not pace), 172 bpm. My spectator spotter and compadres who volunteered to tell me my position after the bike yelled dismal words: fourth place. But I wasn't surprised. The lead woman in my age division had a 25 minute lead at the beginning of the 26.2 mile marathon run, and I had another three and a half hours of running to the finish line.

That, too, was part of the game plan. I hoped that having done a smart bike leg at a steady heart rate of 155–160 bpm, I still would have the leg strength left to catch and pass my competition in the run. At 172 bpm, I ran down third place, then second place, and at the half way point, 13.2 miles, the first place woman still had a ten minute lead. That was almost a minute per mile faster that I would have to run to catch her before the finish.

The run at the Ironman-Hawaii is a convoluted course that includes a loop off to the side. But, overall, it is basically an "out and back." While I ran the out leg, the lead woman in our age division was on the return leg. I had the opportunity to see her running towards home, the finish line, as she passed me.

Just like in my mental video tape, she looked fried. It's typical of this ultra-distance race. Without a tool to control the pace, a heart rate monitor, the mind gets wild, and the body pays the price for going too fast, too hard, too soon. It's usually the bike that destroys the body and its fuel system. It's always during the run when the triathlete pays the price for the bike.

By mile 21 on the 100+ degree heat of the marathon course, I started letting my mind creep away into negative land: "Did she re-energize? Did she see me and get so motivated that she was able to pick up the pace and suffer more?" I didn't know. I became disheartened. I started to listen to my negative mind chatter. Maybe my plan was flawed, maybe the script I wrote for my video had the wrong ending. Maybe I'd lose.

I looked at my heart rate monitor; it said 155. I was letting my mind allow my body to slow down. I was psychologically beating myself up. I then reached down to that place of confidence deep inside me, way deep, and I picked up my stride. It was painful, extremely difficult. I looked at my heart rate monitor; it read 172. I was able to mentally take it back up.

By mile 22, I saw her. She was running, slowly. I came up quickly from behind and as I passed I said: "Do your best. I'm a master, too." I just couldn't pass her and not acknowledge that I knew who she was or not encourage her. I think what goes around, comes around and that if I play win-win, then my competitors will do well, and I will do well. I looked down at my heart rate monitor: 180.

I stopped looking at my heart rate monitor as I came upon the last half mile of the race. The sun was almost set, the crowds were enormous, and it didn't matter because the adrenal hormones were out of control as probably was my heart rate. I didn't want to know, that's how exciting it is at those moments, after 11 hours of racing in those conditions.

I did it, I won. The mental video tape was flawless. The heart rate monitor—my friend—guided me to the win. It allowed me to monitor the status of my mental attitude and physical stamina, to control it and coax myself towards victory.

My training partner and Fleet Feet Vice President, Syd Winlock, was still out on the course. It was his first Ironman distance race. He had programmed in to race at 145–150 on the bike, and 155 on the run. He sent word ahead for me to relax and get a massage, because he said he would finish two hours behind. He did. He too had coached himself towards a personal accomplishment that he had only dreamt of a year ago. After training with him for months and watching him build his self-confidence, I stood very proudly as he came across the finish line.

Some might say, "Sally, you're 44 years old—why do you care anymore about the finish time, your heart rate, the other woman, a trophy?" You might as well ask Captain Ahab about Moby Dick.

The only way to understand that kind of mentality, that kind of raw drive, is to experience it for yourself. You'll never find true understanding by reading about experiences or how things should be done. Go do it. Go out and train and race and sweat and bleed. Go feel what it's like to reach so deeply inside that you brush against your core Self. Go win and go lose, but never stop learning about the world and about yourself.

It's not about status, awards, media coverage, or money. For me, it's about feeling alive in every muscle of my body and every corner of my mind. It's about that final finish line in life and crossing it with the words "You Did Your Best" inscribed on the finish banner.

Kahlil Gibran in The Beauty of Life wrote "I would not exchange the laughter of my heart...for the fortunes of the multitude." He was so right. My most important personal possessions are my sense of personal fulfillment and my health. I not only recommend them both to you, I recommend that you invest all you've got in their achievement.

Your investment into your health—the knowledge investment (this book), the gear investment (a heart rate monitor), the time investment (your training)—has a personal return that Gibran calls the "laughter of the heart." That is what a heart rate monitor can provide you with—a way to not only achieve better health, but to enjoy it as well. It is a way to live a longer and happier life. And for me, it is the way to feel alive, to feel full and fulfilled. It's not a way of life, it's a way of living.

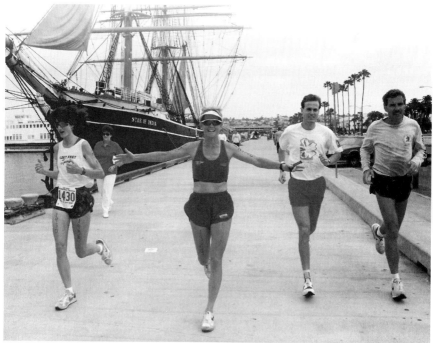

Holding her monitor in her hand, Sally Edwards finishes a triahtlon with three friends. Ultimately, living a longer and happier life is best with friends.

APPENDIX A

HEART RATE FORMULAS

It sometimes seems that there are just as many different calculations for determining training heart rate levels (THRs, also known as your exercising heart rate range or your target heart rate range) as there are different ways of describing heart rates. Following are a number of these ways, but please note that the range of calculation varies dramatically among them, because each of the formulas are dependent upon different parameters. For our purposes, we shall use the profile of an individual who is 35 years old, with a maximum heart rate (MHR) of 180 bpm, a resting heart rate (RHR) of 80, and a heart rate reserve (HRR) of 100.

Karvonen Formula: This method uses the HRR to help find the THR.

$$THR = RHR + \{(MHR - RHR) \times \% \text{ of intensity}\}$$

or

$$THR = RHR + (HRR \times \% \text{ of intensity})$$

So, the THR for a 70% of max training intensity would be figured out as follows:

$$\text{THR} = 80 + (100 \times 0.70)$$
$$= 150 \text{ bpm}$$

Ball State University Formula:

Researchers at this University found that the Age Adjusted Formula often under predicts MHR for older individuals and over predicts for younger individuals. Here's their suggestion:

MHR for women $= 209 - (0.7)$ (age)
MHR for men $= 214 - (0.8)$ (age)

Max HR Method: This method simply uses your unmodified MHR to determine your THR.

$$\text{THR} = \text{MHR} \times \% \text{ Intensity}$$
$$\text{THR} = 180 \times 0.70$$
$$= 126 \text{ bpm}$$

Age-adjusted Method: This method uses your age and your mathematically calculated MHR to determine your THR.

(Warning: Since this method uses a mathematically calculated MHR, not a fitness test determined MHR, the error in this calculation can as high as 40 bpm.)

$$\text{THR} = \text{Age-adjusted MHR} \times \% \text{ Intensity}$$
$$\text{THR} = (220 - \text{age}) \times \% \text{ Intensity}$$
$$= (220 - 35) \times 0.70$$
$$= 185 \times 0.70$$
$$= 129.5 \text{ bpm}$$

As you can see, there is a large range of differences among the above 70% training intensity figures, so consider yourself warned that mathematical formulas may not always be 100% accurate. Following are a few more mathematical formulas to determine different training intensities and other related figures.

Recovery Heart Rate: This is usually determined simply by noting the heart rate after a set post-exercise rest interval, such as two minutes.

Perceived Exertion Method

Rather than use a formula, another way to determine heart rate intensities is by "perceived exertion," that is, how you feel about the intensity. A formalized system for measuring perceived exertion called RPE (rating perceived exertion) was developed by Gunnar Borg, at the University of Stockholm in the early 1980's, and is called the Borg Scale. The Borg scale

Rating of Perceived Exertions (RPE)

RPE	Description very very light	Intensity level Equivalent	Heart Rate Equivalent
6-8			80 bpm
9	very light		90 bpm
10			100 bpm
11	fairly light		110 bpm
12		60% MHR	120 bpm
13	somewhat hard		130 bpm
14		70% MHR	140 bpm
15	hard		150 bpm
16		80% MHR	160 bpm
17			170 bpm
18		90% MHR	180 bpm
19			190 bpm
20			200 bpm

simply quantifies exercise intensity by noting the perceived feelings of fatigue and is obviously not very exact. Perceived exertion is actually how most of us trained before we had heart rate monitors, and this method can still be used when we don't have a heart rate monitor around or when we decide to train by pace monitoring.

The Borg scale runs from 6 to 20. To calculate your training heart rate at any given point, simply add a zero behind your scale number. That is, if the person training says they feel that the workout was hard and gives it a rating of 15, then you would add a zero to the rating, giving an equivalency of a 150 bpm intensity level. This method is called the "No Formula" fitness method.

The Borg formula becomes more inaccurate with increases in age or lack of conditioning. To many beginners, an easy workout of a 10 might be perceived as a 15, causing a considerable discrepancy in determining equivalent heart rates. With time though, someone who uses the no formula fitness scale learns intuitively whether they are exercising at a "light" 10 or a "somewhat hard" 13. The scale is fairly accurate at the high end but is less dependable on the low side, since the differences between a "very light" 9 and a "light" 11 are just too subtle to gauge accurately.

APPENDIX B

MAX HR AND MAX VO2 CORRELATIONS

Thanks to the help of Luc Léger, of the University of Montreal formula's have been designed to show the direct relationship or the correlation between your different heart rate percentages and those of the same for oxygen uptake. In order to improve your maximal aerobic power which is expressed as your Max VO2, your training should be designed to increase this function which is the equivalent of 50-85% of your Max VO2.

But, it is almost impossible to measure this when you are training if you don´t have sophisticated laboratory testing equipment. In the practical world, we train at a percentage of our Max HR not our Max VO2. But since there is not a one-to-one ratio between the two you cannot train at 50-85% of your Max HR and think that you are training your aerobic power.

This is obvious. As explained in Chapter Five, let´s imagine that you are sitting in a chair at rest. Let´s take your resting heart rate, it´s 60 bpm. You took a Max HR test running and you found out that your maximum heart rate for running is 180 bpm. At complete rest, you are working at 30% of your Max HR. If we were to measure your VO2 at this same time resting heart rate it would be about 3.5 ml km - 1min-1 which is about 10% of your max VO2. That is, at rest you are using about 10% of your Max VO2 while you work at 30% of your Max HR.

But, according to Léger, there is a simple formula that will help you correlated one with the other. He found that the percentage of Max HR that corresponds to any percentage of Max VO2 is as follows.

Percentage of Max HR = 38.35 + 0.643 percentage of Max VO2

Unfortunately, Léger with time even developed a better formula with less random variation and less systematic error when he added two key variables to the equation: your sex and your age. Here´s that more accurate calculation:

Percentage of Max HR = 44.6 + 0.57 percentage of max VO2 - 0.41 (your age) + 1.55 sex (females = 2 and males = 1) + 0.0038 Max VO2 x (your age).

You might want to read further here so let me refer you directly to the source if you have more questions. Here are two excellent sources:

1) Ricart-Aquiree, R.M., Léger, L., Massicotte, D. (1990) Problèmes théoriques et pratiques de la prèdiction de la VO2 max. Sciences et sports, 5:143-153.
2) Léger, L., Guitierrez A., Chonière, D., Ricart, R.M., La relation % FC max - % VO2 max en fonction de l´âgee, du sexe et de l´ergomètre. Sciences et Sports 6 (1): 65 (Abstract).

ABOUT THE AUTHOR

Active and athletic from chidhood on, Sally Edwards has championed fitness all her adult life. A competitive runner for more than two decades, she has won races at distances from one mile to 100, and in 1984 she competed in the Olympic Marathon Trails.

No single-sport specialists, Sally Edwards pioneered women's and men's participation in the sport of triathlon. Having completed sixteen Ironman triathlons around the globe, she is the former master's world record of 10 hours and 42 minutes. In all sixteen competitions, she has finished in the top five in either the open/professional or the master's division.

Sally is deeply involved with the promotion and governance of sports in America. She is one of the founders of Triathlon Federation/USA, the national governing body of triathlon in the United States and served as its first Vice-President. She is currently a trustee and an officer if the Women's Sports Foundation, the non-profit foundation dedicated to the growth of girls and women through sports. She is also on the editorial board of Triathlete Magazine and has written for Runner's World, Women's Sports and Fitness, and Triathlete Magazine, as well as for a half-dozen newspapers around the country. She is a well-known public speaker and is the national spokesperson for the Danskin Women's Triathlon Series.

Sally holds double master's degrees, earning her first graduate degree in exercise physiology from the University of California in 1970, then, in 1986, completing a master's in business administration at National University. In 1976 she co-founded FLEET FEET SPORTS, a fast-growing franchise goods chain of 40 stores which are recognized as the premier sports shops for the fitness participant in the United States. In 1992, the Sacramento Chamber of Commerce awarded Edwards the small Businessperson of the Year award.

As she says in The Heart Rate Monitor Book, "Fitness is not just a way of life, it is a way of living."

BOOKS BY SALLY EDWARDS

• The Heart Rate Book

• The Heart Rate Monitor Training Planner and Log**

• Triathlons for Women*

• Triathlons for Kids*

• Triathlons for Fun*

• Heart Zone Training

• Smart Heart, High Performance

• The Triathlon Log**

*To order copies of this book, call or send a check or money order for $10.45 to: Heart Zones, 2636 Fulton Ave., Suite 200, Sacramento, CA 95821 (916) 481-7283, www.heartzone.com

**To order copies of this book, call or send a check or money order for $8.45 to: Heart Zones, 2636 Fulton Ave., Suite 200, Sacramento, CA 95821 (916) 481-7283, www.heartzone.com

All prices include shipping and handling. (916) 481-7283

Sally Edwards publishes The Fitness Monitor Newsletter, dedicated to providing timely, practical information for the competitive athletes, fitness enthusiasts, cardiac rehabilitation patients, personal trainers and others who use heart rate monitors for performance, fitness and health. If you would like to receive a complimentary copy, write to Heart Zones, 2636 Fulton Ave., Suite 200, Sacramento, CA 95821; phone (916) 481-7283 fax (916) 481-2213. One-year subscriptions (six issues) are available for $26/year.